Into the Dark
for Gold

Into the Dark for Gold

by Les Rhodes

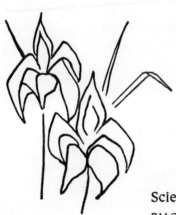

Science and Behavior Books, Inc.
PALO ALTO, CALIFORNIA

Printed in the United States of America

Library of Congress Card 00-133438
ISBN 0-8314-0088-9

Cover design by Jim Marin/Marin Graphics
Editing and interior design by Rain Blockley
Printing by Banta Press

CONTENTS

v

Chapter

FOREWORD

by
J. Linn
Mackey

Lessie Anne asked me to write this foreword from my experience as her husband. I begin with a story that grows out of a recent conversation between us. Lessie Anne was discouraged that day as we sat and talked together in our sunroom. With tears filling her eyes, she said, "I feel so sad for you, J. You didn't expect to have a wife with Parkinson's. This isn't what you signed up for." Those words came from a dark place where hope falters and endurance wanes. These can be dark places for me, as well. I, too, am discouraged at times when I stand by, feeling helpless, as the woman I love suffers.

Why begin with a dark and painful place? It is far from being the whole of my experience in this loving marriage. Still, it is important not to romanticize the situation with which we both live. I want to tell something of my part of the story as honestly as I can. It is what Lessie Anne does in the essays that follow.

When I heard her words of concern, I responded emphatically. "Not true! Not true. Remember? We talked about it all, way back then, early in our relationship." We had been friends for over twenty years before adding romance to friendship. I was well into mid-life. The wonder is that love past mid-life can be as intoxicating and romantic as in one's teens and twenties. That is my experience, anyway. And it includes something more—a wisdom, perhaps, a poignancy, and openness to life arising from the realization that one is looking toward the end of life, not its flowering.

Back together after having been apart, we had spent that long-ago afternoon swept up in romance and passion. Our exchange came at that time when day turns to dusk, before night descends. Perhaps experiencing the dusk symbolically, as a reflection of where I was in life, triggered what followed.

In that close, mellow space of our reunion, I had also felt and tried to give voice to a dark and foreboding presence. "Suppose we marry and I have a heart attack or, even worse, a stroke. You could be stuck with taking care of an invalid. I don't want to saddle you with that."

Lessie Anne also felt the mood. We had both considered death and disability but had not voiced anything with each other. Now, as dusk gathered into darkness, we felt and spoke our deepest fears and, in that voicing, gradually felt relieved and filled with an encompassing compassion that opened the door to deepened intimacy. We pledged to one another: "Even if debilitating illness and death come, so that we have but a brief time together, I choose this relationship and all it may bring with all of my heart and soul."

We had confronted the dark. In the spring of our love, which was also the autumn of our lives, the cosmos had brought us face to face with the great archetypes of illness and death. As the ensuing essays show, in every beginning is also an ending, and in each dusk is the promise of a new dawn: light and dark, life and death—intertwined, interconnected, inseparable. Again and again, we renew those words from our hearts as we live into the destiny of our pledge, experiencing all the feelings of which the human heart is capable.

Sometimes anger wells up within me. How could the universe visit this on my beloved? How cruel to limit and pain this wondrous, life-filled woman! I am angry that illness has come too soon, too soon after I have realized this relationship, which I dreamed about and longed for so many years of my life.

When I wake from sleep in the dark of night and the forces of life are at their nadir, grief waits for me. I have even experienced Parkinson's as a suitor with whom I compete for the affection, interest, and attention of the woman I love. Even with all my ardor and effort, she first must listen to and attend to Parkinson's needs and demands.

It has taken me ten years and much inner work to say, ". . . not my will, but Thine." I am learning that I can accept this as our lot, our task in the midst of deep personal pain. This is the journey we are called to make. Sometimes, I am aware that companioning Lessie Anne on this journey with patience, courage, and love is the best thing I will do in this life. Others may reach places of fame and fortune that I will never reach, but no one else can companion my beloved on this journey as well as I.

Enough of the dark. I want to speak of the light, of the gold in this journey we share. Medical science has provided medication that, when it reaches the proper level, allows Lessie Anne to function with near normalcy. She continues her practice. We go about our lives pretty much as we would without Parkinson's. Medication allows us to live an active social life, to travel, to attend conferences, to ride bicycles, and to go sailing with friends on the inland waterway and even the Caribbean. For stretches of time, I am hardly aware of our Parkinson's companion.

An equally important contribution to the quality of our lives is Lessie Anne's attitude and spirit. She is usually strong, vibrant, hopeful, and positive. It is not that she does not feel the dark, even enter the dark. Rather, it is because she can experience her dark despair so fully, so vulnerably and courageously, that she finds nuggets of gold, gleanings of meaning, which she brings back to renew her life with positive energy and purpose. Because Lessie Anne enters the dark, both of our lives are deeper, fuller, and richer.

After she makes a descent, after the gestation, and after her writing process, we sit together in our sunroom while she reads me her tales of dark and gold. As deep emotions well up within me, in both of us, tears often flow between us. At those times, we enter a holy space that extends throughout this world and beyond.

Lessie Anne has shown me that the spirit's journey into the crucible of illness can reach depth and meaning that partakes of timeless significance. Without Parkinson's, we might never have taken such a journey or found this space of timeless significance. And because of this journey, everything is transformed.

This book speaks to these journeys, the suffering soul's descents into the dark, and the gold found there. These essays invite us into the realm of the soul's darkness, depth, and discovery.

ACKNOWLEDGMENTS

This book is dedicated to my parents, Lela and Abie Rhodes, who have given me life over and over and over again; to J. Linn, the beloved of my heart, who explores the soul-filled heights and depths of love with me; and to our young adult children: David King, Tanya King, Karee Teague, Alisha Mackey-Wilson, Craig Poplars, Michael Teague, Scott Wilson, Jonathan Teague, and Jacob Wilson. You teach me how to make room for more joy!

"Sisters" Priscilla Schmitt and Katherine Henderson and "brothers" Carl Schmitt and Chuck Henderson have been loyal witnesses to my process. Our family is one in which love is readily available.

From a wellspring of care, friends and colleagues have nourished me in this very personal project.

I want to thank Bob Spitzer and Rain Blockley of Science and Behavior Books for their faith in me, for their patience with me, and for the three little words that have changed my life: "go for contract." My editor, Rain, has crawled into my brain and brilliantly fine-tuned what within my depths yearned to be expressed. She understands I write because I must.

Special appreciation goes to author Rick Herrick, who recognized the writer in me even before I did; and to editor Susan Snowden for her guidance and encouragement in the initial stages of putting my story out in the world.

Talking about what matters and listening devotedly, my Salon group is a community of important nourishment in my life. I thank each member for bearing with me and for often finding celebration in the gravest of situations. Zoe Racey of Salon transformed every word in my first draft of longhand twists and turns into computer elegance. This book could not have been born without her skill and optimism.

To those dear friends who, with tears and tenderness, have listened to me read my essays, I give thanks: Belinda Novik, Posie Dauphine, Pat Webster, Bill Thorp, Laurie Percival-Oates, Lynn Jaffe, and John Hartley. Also Jean McLendon, Judith Wagner, and Margarita Suarez—all from Avanta, the Virginia Satir network.

Jungian Diplomate Lois Harvey has shepherded me on this journey with compassion, unflinching courage, meaningful insights, and deep wisdom. She is a blessing in my life.

And to my clients over the past twenty-five years, I express openhearted gratitude for the opportunity to share in a part of your life journeys. You have taught me so much about suffering the dark to find the light.

And to you the reader, you hear me into song.

> Lift every voice and sing till earth and heaven
>   ring—
> Ring with the harmonies of liberty.
> Let our rejoicing rise high as the listening skies;
> Let it resound loud as the rolling sea.*

---

*Lift Every Voice and Sing," *The Presbyterian Hymnal* (1990),
p. 563.

INTRODUCTION

Winter's stillness drew me into my depths like a bear who lumbers into deep retreat that life may be given again. A cold moon ruled the sky, the ridges, and the gorges of these durable old Appalachian mountains where I live. Naked down to their bones, trees shook eerily, like graveyard skeletons dancing to the rhythm of the wind. After the wind came blizzards to bury all that moved in these mountains, until silence covered the earth. There would be many frigid nights like this before springtime tugged once more at the dormant roots and bulbs in my yard.

Eventually, we each encounter some event that brings us to peer into a deep and mysterious chasm within ourselves that we know we must explore. In the winter of my fifty-first year, in 1991, I was diagnosed with young-onset Parkinson's Disease. Thus began a personal descent into the dark and fearsome places within me so that life may be given again.

Stillness was not easy for me that winter. I felt called by the forces-that-be to begin my own down-going to find meaning in my illness. Illness and death are archetypal patterns from which I tell the story of my experience with chronic illness because in the telling my heart opens and my life expands.

Although this book deals with my process around my condition, I intended it to speak to any who struggle with adversity and long to transform personal sorrow and pain into a process of spiritual growth. Telling the truth of my life story defines who I am now and expands my connection to others. While the context of your and my stories are different, the longings of our hearts and spirits are more alike than not. When you know my heart and I know yours, the rest are mere details.

Having Parkinson's means my brain chemistry does not reliably ensure normal flexibility and movement. Although this illness manifests differently with each person, symptoms may include muscular stiffness and rigidity, imbalance, tremor, fatigue, and contraction of muscles even at rest. Parkinson's is progressive (gets worse) over time. Untreated, its symptoms become increasingly severe or degenerative. It may be disabling, debilitating, and potentially devastating, as I witnessed with my grandfather when I was a girl. Even today, the stories we do not want to hear concern those patients shuffling through their remaining days and years in nursing homes. Their agony pierces my heart.

As yet, no cure exists for this condition, although research is heartening. Pharmaceutical treatment benefits many of us. Others find it difficult to manage side effects of medication: involuntary and erratic movement of muscles known as *dyskinesia*. These gestures may be awkward or flowing. That is a frequent aspect with which I contend. From time to time, a total stranger has asked me if I am a dancer. The first time it happened, I was browsing in a bookstore. As I stood at the bookshelves, my body swaying subtly, I was startled to hear the voice of a young man next to me, "I have been watching you," he said. "You must be a dancer. You are so graceful." Of course, he had no way of knowing how much his compliment meant to me.

Periodically, newspapers and television programs report new surgical procedures, more effective medications, and many diverse approaches for contending with the illness. Writers often refer to Parkinson's as the "little darling of neurology" and the 1990s as the "decade of the brain."

Parkinson's produces no infection or inflammation that challenges the immune system. Rather, the *substantia nigra* of the brain, the area that controls movement, has insufficient levels of an amino acid called *dopamine.* This chemical regulates normal flexibility and movement, the major deficits in Parkinson's. Since the immune system is not under attack, that allows those of us in the Parkinson's community to differentiate ourselves from those with life-threatening illnesses and thus maintain our tenuous grasp on health and hope.

The cause of Parkinson's is unknown. Some evidence supports the theory that responsibility may lie with environmental poisoning (insecticides, anesthesia, and possibly even well water). Only recently, scientists identified a defective gene in some Parkinson patients, adding genetic predisposition to its possible etiology.

Probably the most dramatic discovery for Parkinson's and many other health conditions is stem cell research, which isolates and grows the parent cells of all cells hopefully making it possible in time to replace brain cells.

Science offers me facts—significant evidence in measuring and evaluating what I can know through my senses. Research findings and empirical evidence are important aids to understanding the ongoing adversity in my life, but they omit the personal specifics of its context. What of my psychological patterns? What of the questions of my soul? What process of life events connects Parkinson's to my past, even to earlier generations? And what of the questions lurking in the shadows of childhood fears: Why me? What have I done to deserve this?

"We are poisoning our own families, our people, with environmental chemicals," my doctor commented as we scanned my life history for chemical toxicity. In terms of scientific validity, we have yet to prove what causes Parkinson's. In terms of my deep knowing and likely evidence from the laboratory, however, my illness connects with two early experiences. In 1944, when I was five, my doctor recommended removing my tonsils to reduce the frequency of colds. This happened with many kindergartners back then.

In those days, the standard anesthesia for a child's tonsillectomy was half a can of ether. It took three and a half cans (seven times more than the usual amount) to override my body's protest. I screamed and fought against hospital attendants who pinned my wrists and ankles as I floated in and out of consciousness. My body knew ether was an enemy, and I nearly died from the extreme dose.

Upon completing the operation, the surgeon told my parents that I was "allergic to ether" and should never be exposed to it again. When my mother asked why he had not stopped the operation, the surgeon replied, "We had to finish!" For hours, the anesthesiologist sat at my bedside, patting my body in the rhythm of a normal heartbeat. Later, when I returned to consciousness, I curled up in a little ball beneath the hospital blankets. "If I can make myself small enough and keep my eyes closed tightly," I remember thinking, "maybe the people wearing white clothes won't see me." My mother and father wisely requested that I be released to the familiarity and safety of our home, where I quickly recovered.

Forty years later, I began manifesting symptoms as a consequence of this patriarchal error in judgment about getting the job done no matter the cost. At that time, almost all surgical protocols called for ether as a general anesthetic, despite its potential for serious (and not uncommon) side effects. Looking back, I believe the ether overdose knocked out a substantial number of my brain's dopamine-producing cells. What a heavy price for curing a cold!

Until my diagnosis of Parkinson's, I did not know the facts of my tonsillectomy. Initially, I felt relief at learning of the ether overdose. It offered counterbalance for the comments of well-intended friends and relatives who saw me as creating my own reality, even bringing this condition upon myself. If I just had enough faith, I would be healed. I had also struggled painfully at first with the notion that God was punishing me for infractions that exiled me from grace.

I have since come to understand that my contributions to my illness comprise the ways I have betrayed my own nature—my own unique pace and style of living in the world—with competition and striving for recognition in the world. Like my doctors, I had wanted to get the job done. Excel! Achieve! Perform!

The trauma of my tonsillectomy compounded another event of the previous year. Sick with a high fever, I was upstairs in bed awaiting the doctor. He would make me well, my mother promised. I waited and waited for what seemed like a very long time. Finally, he arrived at the kitchen door, his booming voice filling our house.

Why were he and my parents taking so long? I worried. They're talking and talking, and I'm up here all by myself, sick! At last, I heard their footsteps on the stairs. "Well, shall we let her live or not?" asked our doctor in his big voice. My parents laughed and laughed.

To the literal mind and intuitive sensitivity of a four-year-old child, however, this was no laughing matter. In that instant, I dropped into a black and lonely space. With shock, I concluded I was not safe. My parents were laughing about my life. They might actually let me die.

Within my four-year-old powers of reasoning, this was an emotional atrocity. I had overheard what they *really* thought. It was up to me to take care of myself. I would find the button that could turn off my heart when I was endangered. That way I wouldn't be hurt.

Sadly, I did not talk with my mother or father about what I heard or the meaning I placed on it. Until I was in my late teens, no one witnessed my despair as, from time to time in a mostly happy childhood, that dark and deep loneliness sneaked back to clutch my heart. Fortunately, when I finally told my mother, she expressed shock and sorrow, then reassured me of her protection and love. Today, that lonely space is a well-healed scar, leaving only a tiny dark cave in my heart.

Meanwhile, seeds of anger at patriarchal authority found soil in those four- and five-year-old traumas. They sprouted and grew over the years in many life contexts before presenting their ailing foliage for healing in my spiritual crisis as a middle-aged woman.

Parkinson's is becoming more and more familiar as public figures such as Michael J. Fox, Muhammed Ali, Billy Graham, Janet Reno, Katharine Hepburn, and even the Pope reveal their own struggles with the condition. These people seem to acknowledge their limitations openly so that they can live a life of balance as they participate on the world stage. I have great respect for the honesty and bravery of all of us who are living whole lives without pretending we have no disability or trivializing our struggle. Pulling off a performance that seeks to conceal it from others splits the psyche. I know. I tried—and sometimes still try—to deny and hide my muscular stiffness and my left foot's kick and limp. It traps my own energy in deceit. I cannot afford to waste my life's energy in pretense.

While I cannot mobilize power over my limitations, I can and do express my capabilities within those limitations. My reality is that chronic illness has elected me, for its own enigmatic purpose, and I must find a way to live into whatever meaning I make of that purpose. I would surely despair of a life devoid of meaning and purpose.

In the thinking of my mentor, Virginia Satir, we have a need to make sense of the information we take into ourselves through our senses. Automatically, we put meanings or interpretations on what we see, hear, touch, smell, and taste. Meanings stimulate feelings, and feelings attach to self-worth and finally result in influencing our behavior. The challenge is to face and contemplate how my illness is healing me. This is my sacred work. I call it a holy passage, a spiritual journey that takes me off the well-beaten path into unknown territories of my inner life.

"Reach into the darkness to bring forth the golden bough," Jungian analyst Lois Harvey has gently and persistently nudged me over the years.* Her presence in my life is a blessing as she shines soft light on the pathway of healing. And so it is that I travel my spiritual journey in more intentional ways now, growing deeper instead of broader as I explore the wastelands, the cliffs,

---

*Personal conversation, 1992.

and the chasms of my psyche that imperil life's terrain when health diminishes.

Plummeted about by waves of disbelief and sorrowing, surprise and fear that rolled over me after my diagnosis, I nearly missed hearing an almost inaudible inner voice calling to me from my depths. After seeing my doctor, J. and I got ice cream cones and sat in silence as we ate. I listened deeply to this voice, which seemed both winin me and outside me. The message was clear: "Now you can do what you want to do—not every now and then, but every day. Your life requires this."

Instantly, I felt the tightness in my body soften and begin to drain from me. With that release, I became aware of feeling liberated from expectations I had placed on myself to earn my father's love and to live out my mother's dreams through extraordinary performance.

"Do what you love. Find your ownn song and sing it," the quiet voice insisted.

Learning to live with an ongoing illness would text me in every way. This tale of my spiritual journeying draws on evocative material from the challenges and cherishings of personal relationships and the symbolic life of the spirit that enriches ordinary tasks. It draws on archetypal—that is, universal—themes embedded in mythology, transformative images, the application of active imagination, and dreams from my unconscious. These dreams appear in the text under the heading "Dreamlights." They are all significant for integrating

Parkinson's into not only my activities but also my very being. I am reluctantly learning to befriend this illness.

Lying on the earth in the thick soft grass of my back yard was soothing for me at five years old. At fifty-five and beyond, it still is. This book tells of my descents and my emergings, which renew the memory of who I am called to be. These callings of the soul have plunged me into deepened awareness in which the feminine side of God—woman, earth, and goddess—emerges in consciousness. Certainly, Parkinson's affects what I *do* in my life and the roles I play. More importantly, however, who I *am* as a woman with a chronic health challenge is a process of continual transformation. I think of myself as a well person with a chronic illness.

LOSS

From the runway gate, I had a clear view down the long corridor to the 747 that would take Tanya, my daughter, to her beloved Craig, awaiting her arrival in England. She was the last to board, and I knew she would not look back. We had already talked about that. Still, I wanted to call out, "Wait, stay a little longer. Must there be an ocean between us?"

I knew the answer. She was ready to give birth to herself, to create an identity that would reflect not mine, but her own nature. I told myself that she had gotten enough of what she needed from me to take this next step into the world. But in this moment of separating, I grieved silently. What have I done, I wondered. Have I raised my children to break my heart and leave me? Is that what life requires? Soon, all I could see was Tanya's backpack bulging beneath a cascade of long blond hair that swayed with the assurance of a young woman resolved. And I knew life requires precisely this.

While Tanya was setting out on her own journey, my son David was leaving the mountains to begin a new life in Charlotte. He was also moving through his own identity transition. A natural athlete from the time he was eight years old, David excelled in college sports only to discover that beneath his linebacker brawn resided a lean and sensitive poet who would in time write songs and poems and develop social skills for communicating with people of wide diversity.

I was in the process of closing my private practice for a six-month absence while J. Linn was packing our house for rental. We would miss terribly his two young adult daughters, Karee and Alisha. They would stay in North Carolina and join us in New York for adventuring. J. would be directing the Appalachian State Loft in New York City while I sought physicians and healers who might help me. We hoped the time away would offer us an opportunity for rejuvenation, which we both needed, and enable us to find answers to questions regarding my health. In the midst of these life changes, before my diagnosis, I had a dream—a dream that seemed prophetic and more emotionally charged than any dream I can remember. It was late Fall of 1990.

Dreamlight 1990

I dream of two purple irises planted in the earth, their buds pregnant with creation's vitality, sword-like foliage protectively encircling blossoms unfurled by the sun's gentle touch. With imperial grace, they stand rooted in the Great Mother, the Dark Goddess of Earth, from whom all things are born and to whom all must return. And I am infused with love for her creation.

Suddenly, without warning, a brutal force rips blossoms, bulbs, roots, and foliage from the earth's fleshy lap, leaving a jagged and deep lesion vulnerable and unprotected. I shift instantly from observer to participant, as the earth's silent wails become my own. In my dream, I embody this Great Mother, the living Gaia, our fertile soil violated, our souls stricken with grief at the loss of our body's fruit. Her grief, my grief, the grief of all souls unite us as one—woman, mother, Earth—in a vessel of sorrows, where love is a scream of anguish and compassion a shared despair. Confused and afraid, we peer into a gaping wound as I awaken, weeping with deep sorrow.

This dream seemed to be about the loss of my children to life's inevitable summons and my own loss of identity as mother. I had no one now to mother. The message was harsh. On waking, my sorrow seemed linked to a deep and eminent loss. Rather than abating after a good cry for my children, my feelings intensified as I was drawn into the dream's ambience. I was amazed feeling such vivid identification with the Earth Mother. Who and what is this maternal presence? Where did she come from? And what does she want of me, I wondered. Clearly, she was a powerful presence—indeed, a holy figure. I felt bonded to her and through her to a great feminine principle that seemed to be leading me deeper into Earth to find my soul.

This sacred figure I knew was a goddess. Perhaps she was a manifestation of the Black Madonna, a way of naming an aspect in my own psychology that has not yet been developed. Perhaps she was called Sophia:

archetype of the divine feminine. In her wisdom, she would come to lead me more deeply into Earth to discover and to feel the vulnerability of my wound. There I would meet my soul. The presence of this wounded dark mother brought me comfort as she and I joined in anguish that echoes the cries of Christ's passion: *my God, my God why have you turned your back to me.*

This dream would soon unfold its meaning for my life. It would become a call to wake up and transform my life.

DIAGNOSIS

This chapter describes the process that led to my diagnosis of young-onset Parkinson's. As you will see this was not simple or straightforward. No direct medical test identifies Parkinson's. The process spanned years and involved my intuitions and dreams.

The brightness of the morning sun poured through the skylight in my office creating a fanciful dance between refracted sunshine and a large crystal hanging from the ceiling. The crystal had been a gift from my dear J. Linn. We had married a year earlier in the fall of 1986, and I was beginning to feel the wear of commuting between my closing practice in Chapel Hill and my growing practice in Boone. Rocking in my favorite chair, I was counseling a couple in my Chapel Hill office in 1987 when an unusual flutter rippled over the top of my left foot. As it was unlike any sensation I had felt before, I paid attention. After the session ended, I held my foot in my hands, troubled by the vulnerability I felt as the flutters persisted uncontrollably. My mind went to the benign bone tumor that a surgeon had removed from that foot twenty years earlier.

Within three weeks, I saw my family doctor, who referred me to another orthopedic surgeon. It seemed reasonable to assume that the prior surgery had weakened my foot's structure such that daily pressure on the foot was now producing muscular spasms. The surgeon prescribed orthotic supports to wear in my shoes.

Over the next two years, a painful cramp of twisted muscles, little by little, replaced the fluttering in my foot. In addition, a barely discernable vibration, reminiscent of a cat's purr, inhabited my body as my feet and hands began to feel thick, like the consistency of honeycomb. Stress clearly exacerbated these sensations and time passed with subtle changes.

By l989 I was having a difficult time trying to hide my discomfort. It seemed my symptoms worsened daily during the summer of 1989. Having accepted the invitation to be a trainer at Virginia Satir's Avanta-sponsored Process Community, I spent five weeks at this annual training conference in Colorado. This was part of my conscious aspiration: to follow in Virginia's footsteps.

I realize in looking back that while I saw Virginia Satir intermittently, she was influencing my decisions, especially during 1985 through l988, the year she died. Our friendship began in the late seventies when my dear friend and graduate school professor, M'lou Burnett, introduced me to this woman whom people often called the "Christopher Columbus of family therapy." I had already been inspired by M'lou's style of Virginia's work and was eager for training. In January 1980 I joined approximately fifty other therapists and counselors for an intensive month-long seminar whose purpose was to train directly with Virginia in her Growth Model of change and transformation.

Virginia often visited M'lou's home in Springfield, Illinois, for rest and rejuvenation during her trips across the country. As I then lived down the street from M'lou's home, I had opportunities to hang out with both brilliantly creative women. In those intimate, unstructured times, my devotion to and admiration for Virginia grew.

Her exquisite extraversion and my craving for introversion brought us to a point of conflict. I knew she believed in me and nudged me to shine. In 1985 she invited me to be one of the trainers at the annual Process Community. My personal life was in too much flux, I thought, and so I declined.

Having missed that opportunity to be a trainer in 1985, I was determined not to do so in 1989. I knew I was in trouble physically and tried to make a deal with the powers-that-be that if they would help me get through this challenge I would never push my body beyond its limitations.

At the Process Community, the pain in my foot intensified as I pressed on. At night, J. Linn patched me up, comforted me, and renewed me so that I could be "on" the following day. I made it through. Not until our final faculty evaluation session did I break through my overdrive mode and tearfully confess my suffering. I was having trouble tying my shoes, buttoning my blouse, and fixing my hair. Even walking was an effort. It was my dear friend Jean McLendon who noticed I was limping and inquired with sensitivity and care. What a relief to come clean! The loving concern of my supportive colleagues gave impetus to facing my illness and using it to make changes in my life. I began to realize that in the moment what is, is enough. I desperately needed that lesson.

After polio paralyzed Milton Erickson, he regained upper-body movement by visualizing the detailed steps required of his muscles. Remembering this, I discovered I could walk more confidently if I visualized the steps while feeling into the experience of walking—that is, imagining what process my body must go through in order to walk. Even before taking simple steps, I rehearsed my movements, sometimes even singing a tune in my head while matching the rhythm with my feet.

Fear and debility now haunted me. After years of tracking illusive and baffling symptoms, I felt helplessly victimized by this condition. I was also foolishly inflated to think that if only I had a diagnosis with appropriate treatment, I would return to the *status quo ante* of my life—a relentless pursuit of achievement in the world.

Wrong! It did not take long to realize that grandiosity had no place in my life if I wanted to live with quality. Eliminate all stress advised my longtime friend and colleague, psychologist Belinda Novik. It seemed impossible. Every aspect of my life was in transition, and I felt challenged to excel through heroic efforts. After packing my son and daughter off to college, I had moved from the Piedmont to the mountains of North Carolina to remarry. I had also been teaching as adjunct faculty at the university nearby, leading growth groups, presenting workshops, working on a doctoral degree, and maintaining a full-time psychotherapy practice.

Yet I knew Belinda was right. Clearly, my agenda was too much to continue. Simplify! I would need to keep energy flowing in me. That meant expressing thoughts and feelings and resolving problems as they came.

My analyst, Lois Harvey, encouraged me to focus on what I *could* do instead of what I *could not* do. I set about the ongoing process of releasing requirements and obligations, tasks and duties that no longer fit my life and no longer returned energy to me. And as I followed Belinda's and Lois's counsel, a more patient attitude unfolded in me, over time. I listened—*really* listened—to a faint, yet, persistent inner voice that seemed to grow in its wisdom about exactly what adjustments I needed in my life. The enticement of worldly recognition faded as a more immediate presence drew me into moment-by-moment awareness.

One important change was to move my office from downtown Boone to my home in Blowing Rock. There, among the rhododendron of the Appalachian mountains and my lovingly tended flowerbeds, I feel a reunion of body, mind, and spirit in which personal self and professional self are of one weaving.

I found immediate relief and unexpected contentment by reducing the expectations I had placed on myself. I withdrew from my active schedule and found it surprisingly easy to spend hours at a time on the deck of my home while the full-shining sun held me intently in its warmth. All distractions of the day seemed erased by the sun calling me to one piece of life at a time— earth and sky cradling my being in sweet nature on a spring day. Rather than going into a depression, I followed my body's lead and turned my attention inward. I was astonished at how natural I felt surrendering to the peace and serenity of a slower pace in the natural world.

Painstakingly, and with determination, my husband and I continued searching for a diagnosis. Examinations, tests, medical workups, even a Magnetic Resonance Imaging (MRI) scan revealed nothing abnormal. My health appeared fine, and I felt solid internally. Yet my mobility was ebbing rapidly. Terror often gripped me.

As months stretched into years, many valuable contributions to my care came from skilled practitioners: my family doctor, two orthopedic surgeons, two neurologists, a psychiatrist, three physical therapists, two chiropractic physicians, a hypnotherapist, a practitioner of acupuncture, and healers skilled in bodywork, including Rubenfeld Synergy, Feldenkreis, Traeger, massage, and polarity balancing. Some of them are still vital members of my support team. In those days, though, before anyone could diagnose my condition, my particular set of symptoms eventually perplexed each practitioner, who in turn then urged some version of lifestyle change. Surely I must be "exhausted," "depressed," or "burned out," they advised.

With both hope and dread, my husband and I rented our house, packed our bags, and left for his scholarly assignment off campus. I took a leave of absence from all my work. For six months, I struggled against a grinding decline with the support of physical therapy exercises three times a day, long stretches of rest, chiropractic work, psychotherapy, and bodywork.

The work of Ilana Rubenfeld—professional musician, gifted psychotherapist, and founder of Rubenfeld Synergy®—made a tremendous impact on me at that time. Her approach was to unite body, mind, and emotions. Her hands *listened* with a finely tuned knowing to discover where my body was holding pain. In that touch, defenses and resistances melted and I felt glimpses of new life beginning to stir within.

The night after my first treatment with Ilana, I dreamed of being encircled and comforted by a grove of lush, full green trees. At my next appointment, I reported my dream image and the comfort I felt with trees surrounding me. Ilana smiled and said "Ilana is the Hebrew word for tree."

Dreamlight
1990

From time to time a disturbing image in my dreams began to appear in the outer environs of my dreamscape.

> An old man, stooped and stiffened, shuffles slowly in the shadowed horizon of my mind's landscape. Like heavy pendulums, his arms hang inertly from his shirtsleeves, his upper body bent low, his shoulders falling down like teardrops. His massive hands shake with metronomic regularity. In the foggy cover of hypnagogic space, between waking and

sleeping, I squint to bring him into sharper view
before the dreamlight swallows him. At times, I
even feel as if I am in his body and he in mine,
our boundaries merging in strange familiarity.

On my return to North Carolina, I immediately
sought out my family doctor, Pat Guiteras, M.D. In
addition to his usual compassion and quietly offered
expertise, he was baffled and grave. "So much is at stake
now, Lessie. What do *you* think is happening to you?"

I was about to respond with my usual frustration
when emotion spontaneously swelled within me. Surely,
some aspect of my psyche had been poised in wait for
this exact question. Sobs filled my throat and tears rolled
down my face as words tumbled out from a place of

deep inner knowing. "I'm not diagnosed. I know something is terribly wrong," I heard myself say.

Suddenly, in a lightning bolt of recognition, I saw the bent old man of my dreams. "My grandfather!" Explaining to my doctor, I continued: "I see him in my dreams. I feel like I'm in his body. Sometimes I even move like he did. He had Parkinson's Disease!"

I saw the stark recognition of truth in my doctor's face, along with much care and concern. There it was. We both knew. In that instant I knew my life would never be the way it had been before.

Another neurological workup by a specialist confirmed my intuitive knowing and my doctor's deductive diagnosis. Parkinson's Disease. Treatable? Yes. No known cure . . . yet.

In the confusion, shock, and even relief of a confirmed diagnosis, my husband's unwavering presence made the strongest impression on me. We often shivered together in one another's arms. His loving body created a safe and strong container for me as the hurt, fear, and anger in my heart poured out through tears. I fed on the nourishment of our souls' strength and our bodies' embraces.

With sensitivity and swift appraisals, my mother and sisters began a search for a specialist. They called the twenty-four-hour hotline service of the Parkinson's Foundation in New York City, which has a register of specialists. Surprisingly, North Carolina showed no Parkinson's specialists registered then. The nearest was Dr. Kathleen Shannon, the physician who directed the Movement Disorders Clinic at Vanderbilt University Medical Center in Nashville, Tennessee.

Close enough. A seven-hour trip to see Dr. Shannon would do just fine. However, nothing could have prepared me adequately for the shock I experienced on approaching the waiting area. Milling about were people with movement disabilities of all description. "I don't belong here!" I wailed silently, refusing to sit among them. Instead, I told the receptionist that I would wait in the nearby Ob-Gyn clinic. (Since that initial visit, I have grown in compassion and now recognize how tenaciously I can hold on to denial.)

I was surprised on meeting Dr. Shannon to discover her to be so young. J. and I guessed she was in her mid thirties. I wondered if she were old enough to be an experienced doctor. That was quickly put to rest as her brilliance and thoroughness prevailed. She took copious notes, asking bundles of questions while writing every word in longhand. I immediately liked her quiet, firm authority. I felt safe, hopeful, and met. I also liked her long earrings that danced from her ears above the crisp white coat of her doctoring vestment. Together we have woven a tapestry of complex pieces to maximize the effectiveness of medication.

Week upon week after that visit, my husband and I waited with hope to see what medication would do. For my grandfather, the disease had eventually devastated his life. His Parkinson's developed before the discovery of L-Dopa, the powerful modern-day drug that increases levels of synthetic dopamine in the brain. As I took my medications in the early days, any shred of false security shattered under recurring waves of grief for him, for my loved ones, and for myself.

IRIS

In retrospect, I am certain unconscious dream material presaged my illness. My previous dream of the purple iris came to me only weeks before my diagnosis was confirmed by neurological tests in February of 1991 and by my response to medication. I now had confirmation that the dream spoke to something

47

in addition to the separation from my children. The terrible disruption and dislocation of the dream now mirrored my diagnosis and its accompanying feelings of devastation. Also, the Divine Feminine was pressing her presence into consciousness through my dream, as if preparing me for a descent into the fearsome darkness of my psyche to reclaim my soul.

Dreamlight 1990

In the words of Marion Woodman, "dreams are ahead of consciousness. They resonate with our weeping spirits that long to join with the divine."*

---

*Addiction to Perfection, p. 85.

I dream of two purple irises planted in the earth, their buds pregnant with creation's vitality, sword-like foliage protectively encircling blossoms unfurled by the sun's gentle touch. With imperial grace, they stand rooted in the Great Mother, the Dark Goddess of Earth, from whom all things are born and to whom all must return. And I am infused with love for her creation.

Suddenly, without warning, a brutal force rips blossoms, bulbs, roots, and foliage from the earth's fleshy lap, leaving a jagged and deep lesion vulnerable and unprotected. I shift instantly from observer to participant, as the earth's silent wails become my own. In my dream, I embody this Great Mother, the living Gaia, our fertile soil violated, our souls stricken with grief at the loss of our body's fruit. Her grief, my grief, the grief of all souls unite us as one—woman, mother, Earth—in a vessel of sorrows . . .. Confused and afraid, we peer into a gaping wound as I awaken, weeping with deep sorrow.

Dreams seem to signify that consciousness demands its birth through the empowered expression of our suffering. We can ride life's energy like a wild and mighty mare, its power banked by the earth, until freedom's limits beckon us to a place where shadows lurk and grief pursues. As the joy of living unites with the pain of its consort, death, we unleash a chasm-deep scream of love and loss. Perhaps illness was the only way the soul could get my undivided attention. Several years later, I found myself understanding, day by day, that embracing my woundedness leads me to the realm of the sacred. There, illness becomes divinity as well as disease. The jagged wound becomes a space of mystery to incubate the love of the Earth Mother, the Mother God.

The dream offers two purple irises, the color of passion. In Latin, that word has dual connotations: one that points to passion's agony, the other to its ecstasy. And so it is with my illness, whose agony of limitation at times completely absorbs my mind and whose ecstasy permeates my senses as I ride the rich sounds of Jesse Norman singing "Amazing grace, how sweet the sound" or melt into a symphony by Brahms. Body and soul rip asunder beneath the brutal force of change that necessarily reaches back to life's chaotic matrix to bring forth a new creation of compassion and love.

This awareness makes all the difference as my body and soul fall under a siege that shakes the foundation of my life. The earth quakes beneath my feet. My muscles tighten to resist erupting tremors at the same moment that my symptoms call me to live into the yet unknown truth of my destiny. In the midst of an ominous presence, the heart's compassion reunites soul and substance. In facing my greatest fears, I find myself in the loving arms of mystery, where soul and iris awaken to their dance.

My diagnosed illness became a religious discipline for me, rooted in sorrow and faithful to the deepest truth in me. Daily I practice contemplating my condition's possible symbolic lessons. I have learned to let my pain guide me toward authentic living, in which the achievements of pride become irrelevant. Healing means growing toward wholeness, and wholeness depends on being radically and most purely myself.

In moving toward my pain with concern for my inner life, I lay claim to human dignity through experience. I honor my feelings by expressing them. That is, I choose to reveal my heart on a personal level and on a transpersonal level that transcends time and space. Through grief, I meet the Dark Goddess. Perhaps she has been waiting all my life, this maternal Shadai, She Who Is, Sophia-Wisdom, LaLoba, Gaia. Her names reflect my longing for eternal nearness, biologically rooted in feminine essence. As names for she who cannot be named, they bring hope that she who loves me in my despair does not perish but brings forth new consciousness from the darkness of eternal chaos. Her power and glory fill my soul as I see the feminine side of God revealed. And darkness transmutes into dawn, as agony into joy.

In Greek mythology, Iris is the goddess of the rainbow. Symbolizing connection, she bears the tension of duality: between heaven and earth, spirit and matter, sickness and health, life and death. Such polarities yearn to become the one. Iris thus also represents a wisdom that unites opposites and makes life whole, bringing archetypal healing into flesh made sacred, and God the Mother made ineffable.

The flower's beauty reminds me of life's victory over death and of death's insistence on claiming life for itself—one implying the existence of the other in the struggle of creative paradox. As I grow into the living of my soul, I become more of the iris: body and soul reach for one another with yearning to unite in love with the one soul to which we all belong.

As I end my years of rejecting peace for public acclaim, tears fall to mourn the loss of who I have known myself to be. The pressure to perform, to compete and excel, to strain for the world's credentials dissolve into expanded grace. Such goals now seem much less significant. I surrender to the spirit of holiness within my illness, hidden like veins of gold in the earth's fleshy darkness. What I have felt is a life sentence I also experience as a gift. The Dark Goddess of Earth calls to me in my body's cells now, and I respond with the longing of my soul. And though my symptoms limit my walk upon this sweet Earth, her dark radiance illuminates my way as the iris of my heart bravely blooms.

Even before my diagnosis, J. Linn and I had committed to a way of life that comes from the richness of our shared inner existences. For many years, we have shared a spiritual path and deep connection to one another and to the sacred earth. J.'s steadfast compassion is a great blessing, and his arms were a refuge as I learned to reach into the dark depths of my psyche, hoping to find purpose in my suffering. In struggling to accept the pain and fear, I had to have *meaning*! I also knew that meaning had to come from within, from the intuition of my soul. What parts and aspects were hidden away, denied, unwanted, and undeveloped? I needed all within me that was durable. As I gathered the fragments of my psyche and my life into my heart, I prayed for a spiritual breakthrough to new levels of understanding.

Long years of psychotherapy, my own and that of my clients, had taught me to find hope's glimmer by amplifying the dark as I turn toward pain in quiet introspection. Over the ensuing months, I discovered a deep pool of quietude within me and with my husband— a pool where suffering was and is suffused with meaning.

It is the dwelling place of the self before the wounds of life's vicissitudes, a realm where life force is pure and Grace unabashedly given and received. A guiding power, present there yet unseen, knows my being and continues to reach with me for life even when consciousness despairs.

Surrendering to the mystery of the dark, I have found myself again and again held in a circle of endless light that connects to a long line of souls who have also known suffering and whose hearts have responded with compassion born of loss. As kindness transforms suffering into the purposeful expression of life and destiny, I am moved by the words of Laura Chester, who sensitively describes, "something gives, as if an old rotten rope [has] finally lost its grip on the pier's post and [we] are released into a greater lake, a wider gentleness."* I have felt held by that wider gentleness in the arms of my children, my husband, my parents, my sisters, and the many other loved ones of my life.

Several years after I met her, Dr. Kathleen Shannon moved to Chicago's Rush Presbyterian–St. Luke's Presbyterian Medical Center, where she teaches, does research, and has clinic hours. Every six months since then, I see my family physician and then make my pilgrimage to Chicago to see Kathleen. Sometimes, when

Lupus Novice, p. 147.

I need reassurance or medication adjustments, she and I schmooze on the phone as well. It works.

Even when faith is fragile, staying with the truth of my feelings moment by moment releases me from futile efforts at controlling my body and emotions to fit the expectations of others. Let go, false images. I have no energy left for pretense.

Liberated, I can glide into a freedom to become more naturally who I am born to be. That is truly the individuation that my mentors, Carl Jung and Virginia Satir, espoused. Our illnesses thus become a process for birthing our most authentic and humble selves. Now, as a woman much closer to sixty than fifty, I freely reveal more of myself through speaking my truth congruently, with less concern about other people's opinions of me and more concern that I use my voice as a woman to speak the wisdom of my years. For me, it is a renewal of life.

In his wise book *Body and Soul: The Other Side of Illness,* Albert Kreinheder challenges us to find the symbolic content of disease.*

> The paradox is that the wound, the illness, is also the treasure. The physical misery gets your attention . . . that's where the treasure is, in the images that come with the symptoms. The symptoms open you up. They literally tear you

---

*Body and Soul, p. 53.

open so that the things you need can flow in.
. . . When you become ill, it is as if you have
been chosen or elected, not as one limited and
crippled, but as one to be healed . . . to a wholeness far beyond your previous so-called health.

In March 1991, I felt new sensations in my feet, like
the gentle fizz of carbonated water. This signified that
my muscles were opening and releasing. In place of
cramping rigidity, I could again begin to feel normal and
move flexibly for at least portions of the day. My
medication (Sinemet) was working! My response to the
medication was the most reliable conformation of my
diagnosis. It felt like a miracle. My life had been given
back to me. I was jubilant and grateful.

With the renewal of my body, more of me participated in this new journey of body and soul destiny. That "more of me" had been forged before diagnosis in the crucible of my disabilities and fear. Ultimately, we cannot override fear. It strips us of pride, falsity, and any veils that conceal our truth. Tears of humiliation bend us low as our defenses crumble and we experience our full vulnerability. Our hearts break wide open.

I soon learned that medication can also bring tormenting side effects, as with most ongoing treatment for chronic illness. Vast contrasts in mobility each day teach me that life does call us to suffer its polarities. Jung challenges us to bear the tension of the opposites as we stand between opposing energies while resisting conquest by either extreme: health and illness, life and death, connection and separation, hope and despair, and even the on/off oscillations of Parkinson's. Sufficient dopamine levels in the body offer life and mobility in the "on" phase. This stands in stark contrast to the times of inadequate dopamine, which brings a sinking rigidity that feels like a creeping death. For me, these phases have been known to switch several times a day. The oscillations pose a choice between engaging in a painful battle of opposing realties or accepting my symptoms. If I can heed Satir's gentle coaxing to come closer, come closer to that which is feared—if I can accept these polarities as part of the illness's overall rhythm—something new emerges from within. It is a different perspective, a fresh attitude, both transcendent and immanent. It feels like a gift of grace.

BEFORE THE PRESENT

I was 13 years old when I discovered I had a voice that wanted to sing. Even now, the occasion is still vivid. After the evening meal in our home came piano practice. This released me from washing dishes to serenading my mother and grandmother nightly as they coaxed me through my keyboard assignments from the kitchen. Setting aside my scales and *arpeggios* one evening, I meandered through a family songbook, stopping to play and sing to myself. But when I sang *because you come to me with naught save love and hold my hand and lift mine eyes above.* I nearly swooned with intensity. Melody and lyrics enticed me to sing with all my adolescent zest and passion.

I sang my heart out that evening. Never before had I felt so free and exhilarated. I was amazed at the sound reverberating in my body and pouring out like a mountain waterfall in spring. My family was surprised to hear such a big sound from a girl so young.

The very next day, Mother took me to our church's choir director, who referred me to a voice teacher for an audition but not before signing me up to sing a solo in church the next Sunday. Within weeks, I enrolled in the preparatory school of the University of Louisville School of Music for keyboard and voice lessons plus music theory and sight reading classes. I loved classical music and learned quickly. Breath and sound flowed effortlessly through every cell of my adolescent body. I felt such rapture that it seemed I was riding the pulse of infinite song. My voice sang me!

Our choir director told me I was a soprano, and the voice teacher suggested that time would turn my voice into a contralto. During prep school, my young heroic spirit fed on the soprano arias of great oratorios. Like the mythical Icarus, I longed to fly. I wanted to sing my soul, and I wanted recognition for my achievements: my place in the sun. Nourishing this dream continued for my next twenty years of study, training, practicing, auditioning, and performing.

Yet something was out of balance from the beginning. I loved to practice—often six hours a day during college, where I majored in music. The strain of competition and performance anxiety plagued me, however. To offset my terror somewhat as a student at Maryville College in Tennessee, I had warm support from faculty and other music majors. Still, I never told anyone how afraid I felt. In those days, all I knew about coping with the stress of performance was to pretend it wasn't happening. No one knew about my nausea, diarrhea, heart palpitations, and fantasies of catastrophe and potential humiliation. To rise above fear, I drew on false poise.

Rather than growing in confidence with experience, more performing, and maturity, I remained the hostage of my inner critics. "You're not really all that good, and you know it," they tormented me. "It's only a matter of time till they find out that you're just a flash in the pan. Then what?" The judgmental accusations droned incessantly, unmercifully: "Who do you think you are anyway? You'll eventually make a fool of yourself."

The emotional cost of performing became such that, after many years, I eventually stopped singing altogether. Young and fragile, I had come to cultural evaluation much too soon. I was not ready to go public with my soul. The voice that once flowed from my heart then withered and slipped into my unconscious.

69

I decided to find a new profession—one that valued down-to-earth realness. Surely that would fit better for me. I would become a psychotherapist. And so I did. Twenty years later, it continues to be a very good choice. I came to love the process of psychotherapy. However, I held tightly to hubris and felt an urgency about meeting the expectations of professors and mentors who believed in me as a therapist. Fulfilling my own need to succeed in the world's eyes, I once again let myself be driven by what Jungian psychology calls *negative animus energy:* an overly aggressive masculine energy of the personality. In my case, this has prodded me to do more, accomplish more, excel more and dazzle the public.

For many years I have been working with this over-functioning, driven energy to learn more about myself

so that I am less vulnerable to the expectations and opinions of those outside myself. This energy in its positive
form is a force that is useful in setting and attaining
goals. In its negative form it is destructive. Even now, I
realize I could become so absorbed in this process of
writing as to work straight through lunch, oblivious to
hunger, need for medication, or rest. By that time, my
body would ache, I would be weakened from lack of food,
and my dopamine-deprived muscles would be tight and
uncomfortable. I would be critical of what I had written.

To push and drive on doesn't get me what I want.
What was joyous now becomes corrosive and negative.
Parkinson's insists: "Slow down, way down, let your
engine idle so that you can listen to your intuitive

wisdom. Decisions will come more easily, and you will be at home in your body and soul."

The struggle is ending between the young masculine achiever and the voice of the wise crone who longs to draw solitude around me like a worn and cozy shawl. That is what I long for and truly want. This wise old woman knows that "excellence isn't destiny."* She also knows that a part of healing is the realization that I am capable of slipping back into addictive dazzle. Remember Icarus. He became so enchanted with the fear and excitement of flying high that he ignored his father's caution to steer clear of the heat of the sun, which melted the wax on his handcrafted wings.

---

*Marty Groder, 1995.

It is my habit to see the big picture when making present or future plans. Whether it is having a dinner party, leading a workshop, or spending a week in the Caribbean sailing with friends, I tend to create a glorious experience in my imagination. Usually the initial excitement has no consideration of the nitty-gritty practicalities required to make the event possible. With my physical needs and changes, it is critical that I stay aware of details all the time. Creative adaptation is required now, whether I am planning a picnic or making love, or both. Imagination is worth cultivating.

After my diagnosis, soaring higher gave way to delving into the darkness. For me, fearing the unknown did not diminish the call to discover and bring forth the gift of my illness. What I found was a voice that speaks from the still point of the deepest realness in me. Aside from grounding me in the earth's feminine energy, it reaches with great tenderness to others who are called to dance with the illusive partner of illness and loss. With gratitude and wonder, I recognize this voice—familiar, yet fresh, ancient, yet newly born—as that of the young singer who fled so many years ago. Her soul-full tones resonate with an inner song of life's joys and sorrows and resound with strength. Rising from the inner source of my authenticity to *be* in the *now* of my life, my voice expresses my truth in written words these days. Yet, as it did in my teen years, that truth still originates in my soul.

One who taught me to confront mystery and to listen for the voice of inner wisdom was Virginia Satir. Through a spiritual lens, she led me to see all life as holy and holistic, a process of interconnecting relationships that innately moves toward growth and wholeness. By being centered—that is, balanced—we can hear the wise voice of the deep self within as we make our way, step by step, through the inevitable, chaotic aspects of conscious change and individuation.

Years of training with Satir began in 1977 when I attended one of her workshops in Chicago. In full stature of her nearly six-foot height, she appeared before 500 of us with grace, humility, and abundant joy. Within minutes, a reverent silence permeated the group.

Overflow participants sat motionless on the floor of the aisles or stood at the rear. She began with centering: "Let your beautiful eyes close. Allow the breath to lead you to your home within. There you can reach deep and down to that place within where you keep the treasure known by your name."

A few seemingly simple words spoken with love and compassion touched my soul's center, an inner space of pure acceptance and deep awareness which I recognized as the place of home in my heart out of which I sang so many years before. Satir's meditation and demonstration work with a family that day was an experience of incredible grace. A door opened for me into a new path of conscious trust in myself and a process of healing in the deepest way. I began to understand an intrinsic relationship between self and holy, between self-expression and wholeness that accompanies life's changing process. Virginia's presence continues to support me although her body left the ways of the earth years ago.

To the systems work of Satir, I bring the complement of Carl Jung's analytic depth psychology of dream work, symbols, myth, and metaphor. Both these masters view the person with deep respect and regard for the innate propensity that seeks growth by bringing together the dichotomies of life. Both their models have enriched my life and work tremendously since the 1970s, as reflected in this book. Years of study in Jungian seminars as well as my own ongoing analysis have opened me to a land rich with symbolic images pressing into consciousness in my own individuation. This self-development process entails becoming more real than right in my life-long quest for an authentic existence.

Carl Jung's depth psychology appeals to me by offering a spiritual dimension that is concerned with ultimate questions about life's meaning and the search for wholeness. Both Satir and Jung believed in the drive to individuate, to become the unique person each of us is meant to be. Both expressed deep and abiding trust that the psyche grows toward wholeness innately. While Satir emphasized the quality of communication with others and with parts of ourselves, Jung turned to the unconscious for symbolic representations of relationship. That is, he saw that we often experience aspects of the self through the language of dreams, images, metaphor, and myth.

I use *psyche* and *soul* interchangeably since *psyche* is Greek for soul. It denotes who we are at the deepest spiritual level. I now elaborate briefly on Jungian terms because I will be using them throughout the book. Many chapters refer to *archetypes*, for instance, which are universal patterns of knowing and behaving. As grandmothering replaces the innocence of my inner maiden, I feel time shoving me into the winter of my life, into the archetype of the sage old woman. This wise old woman symbolically contains the energy of menstrual blood in her body to make wisdom instead of babies. It is she who sits on the curb in her purple dress and red hat.*

Probably the most significant archetype of our time is the *shadow,* or the dark unacknowledged side of the personality. Its components are all the unacceptable or rejected parts and pieces of ourselves. It is full of feelings, behaviors, ideas, potentials, and beliefs we do not know well or find comfortable. The personal shadow is like a trunk that begins collecting its contents early in life, when our caretakers reject various aspects of us they find unacceptable for whatever reason. Some of the parts

---

*Jenny Joseph, *When I Am an Old Woman, I Will Wear Purple,* p. 1.

we once learned to reject and leave undeveloped—such as anger—are aspects of ourselves that we later prize. Shadow energy can be positive if we reclaim and learn how to harness its energy.

Coping with and civilizing our shadow parts is the responsibility of the *ego*. To aid in this, we develop a *persona*, a mask or façade that hides our shadow parts and shows the world an acceptable outer personality. This is what I learned so well in showing a poised, confident woman as I was performing while inside I was terrified.

When it is time to grow, who we are, including the persona, must open to the shadow. Some crisis such as illness destroys our sense of order and well being. The persona can no longer resist the power of the shadow. The life that has been gathering in the unconscious now insists on being reckoned with. When I was forced to recognize the realness of a health crisis and its constriction of my physical capacities, I felt vulnerable to the power of disability and death. I felt compelled, not with morbid curiosity but with radical honesty, to turn toward mystery wherever I found it, especially in the form of death. Death insists we find out all we can about dying. In so doing, I sometimes develop a brotherly or sisterly kinship with it. Who I am including my persona is being recreated.

Again and again, I return to the challenge of harvesting positive animus energy for setting and reaching goals in a graceful way instead of over-functioning with negative animus drive. In large part, this book is about *inflation*—an exaggerated state or experience of augmented, bigger-than-life identity with unrealistic human goals that yearn for peace—and its healing. As a woman, I struggle with balancing my own masculine energy. So, too, a man is challenged to integrate his *anima,* or feminine aspect, so as to relate to people with mutuality and to connect to aspects of his inner life.

In times of stress at the crossroads of two conflicting polarities, a third energy emerges gradually. It is a new possibility or attitude in resolving the struggle between the polarities.

At the center of the psyche resides the self. Its purpose is to balance the whole personality with a sense of completeness that is God within.

This book's essays are songs of healing from my heart. The voice silenced in my youth returns with compassion and new vitality, rising from feminine ground where consciousness includes an emerging wisdom that requires suffering as well as celebration. Giving sound and timbre to my woundedness will, I hope, attend and honor the woundedness in us all. My voice joins a chorus of voices, female and male, that express the spirit's liberty through feminine consciousness, singing and dancing the feelings of love made flesh and soul made whole.

THE BREATH
OF OUR ANCESTORS

We carry the history of our lives in our flesh. In our bones and in our spirits, we carry the sufferings and the glories of our fathers and mothers and all ancestors. In the unconscious of our families, we connect to a long line of kinfolk who stand behind us—one hand in ours, the other extended to preceding generations. Into the depths of time, they whisper our names, linking us across centuries to our origins: the place of beginnings, where masculine and feminine truly unite in Mother and Father God.

I called my grandfather "Big Daddy" and my grandmother "Granny." He was a quiet, gentle man, as introverted as my grandmother was gregarious. As a little girl, I loved to slip quietly into their bedroom in the early morning and watch them snuggle. Sometimes, I crawled in with them. Those were happy times. Even after Parkinson's incapacitated Big Daddy, he and Granny managed to hug and kiss the morning in.

My grandfather was a strong man. Family lore tells of his facing the Ku Klux Klan time and again when they tried to intimidate him for actively supporting the blacks in town who demanded better education for their children. As a child, my mother sometimes woke in the night to hear horses of the Klan thundering down the long driveway. My grandfather stood firm on the porch, shotgun at his side, his conviction uncompromised. The hooded riders circled round and round the house on their horses and then rode off.

I remember Big Daddy more as a disabled older man. Even then, he was a brilliant mathematician. My sister Pris and I made up the longest math problems our young minds could conjure, and his mind outran the calculator every time.

Every other day, my mother or grandmother shaved his prickly beard after he and I played a game of seeing how close I could get to his face and still escape getting tickled by his whiskers. He laughed as we played our little game, despite knowing that laughing took a lot of effort and made his shaking much worse. At other times, having ice cream melt in his mouth while my grand-mother patiently fed him spoonful by spoonful brought vague smiles to his stiffened features. I could tell when he felt a little better because he would sing out "Ghost Riders in the Sky" with a *tremolo* in his voice that matched the tremor in his hands.

Eventually, he became too ill to care for at home and we placed him in a Shriner's "Home for Incurables." My mother said that was the hardest day of her life. Smells, sights, and sounds of his nursing home are etched in my memory as indelibly as the words "Home for

Incurables" carved in the stone archway of the front entrance. I still hear my grandfather's feeble voice calling from the room he shared with seven other disabled men. "Won't somebody help old man Nelson?"

Now he comes to me through an illness we share. What does it mean to welcome his presence from the dead? What does it mean to allow myself to live in my grandfather and he in me? His presence connects me to my destiny. Living into the suffering and the love I share with him means looking into the sorrowing of his eyes and knowing they mirror my own. I know something of his suffering, and he of mine. In the realm of the eternal, we are one. My grandfather is the guide into the mystery of forgiveness and into a holy place where the soul is home in God the father and God the mother. Bud Harris writes that "behind the presence of God stands the archetypal spirit of the father: a distillation of the collective experience of all time."

The father archetype contains the polarity of both the judging, domineering patriarch and the protective strength of a loving father. Awkward and unpracticed, my father and I now seek connection with one another in a softer way than what once seemed patriarchal. A fallen patriarch, my father at eighty-six years is now learning to think with his heart. I discover I long for his spirit, whose eternal essence is untouched by the greed of Alzheimer's.

Reaching through memories, fragments of memories, and holes where memories once were, he now contemplates the pieces of his life. As a boy, he learned to play checkers with the men who gathered around the pot-bellied stove in his father's general store. Today, he is still every bit the champion he was then, long term-memory still accessible for remembering his origins. With uncompromised skill, he continues to find pleasure in playing the accordion, to the rest of the family's delight.

The softness of our connection now reminds me of an early childhood memory of traveling alone with him from Indiana to North Carolina on the train. I can still feel the gentleness with which he tried to brush and plait my hair as my mother did.

91

**Dreamlight
1993**

I dream that my mother and I have entered a house to visit Big Daddy and Granny, who are dying. In their bedroom, we are astonished to discover that they aren't there. Instead, we find them nearby in a large sunken shower stall— quite alive. They smile as the area is bathed in light.

We understand that together they have done a wondrous thing. They have pooled their energies to creep and crawl from their bed to the shower, dragging the mattress with them, so that they can make love one more time. Granny is lying between my grandfather's legs with her head on his belly, grinning with de- light. She is totally bald. A worn rag doll also

92

lies on the mattress. My grandfather sees my mother and me and exclaims with glory, unabashed love, and delight: "Nana! Nana!"

I gaze amazed at what my grandparents have accomplished and at my grandfather's pleasure upon seeing my mother and me. I notice that my grandmother looks like my mother. Granny is happy, loved, and dying well.

This dream places me in the realm of my ancestors and the numinous power of the masculine and feminine *conjunctio*, or union, in which ecstasy opens to transcendent spirit. The dream is bathed in light that shimmers and radiates love. An old relationship between the masculine and feminine in my psyche is dying to make

way for a new birth of masculine and feminine relatedness. Perhaps that is the purpose of my grandfather's
presence through Parkinson's in my life.

As in the account of the stone rolled away from the
tomb of Jesus, my grandparents are not where we expect them to be in the dream. They are not dead. From
under death's threat, they have emerged into life's affir-
mation. Their union has given them sufficient strength
to reach water, in which life begins. The shower stall
represents a miniature universe where transformation
takes place in the joining of masculine and feminine.

Even without hair, my grandmother is radiant, her
outward crowning glory unnecessary for receiving my
grandfather's love. He accepts and cherishes her as she

is. My mother and I are included, even welcomed, into their symbiotic bliss. In dying, their hearts open for love to enter—love that is unconditional and forever and represented by the endless renewal of life.

The generations blur in this dream. My grandmother looks like my mother. The small, obviously well-hugged rag doll indicates that the male–female union is not just a grown-up instinct but a genuine enactment of life. My grandparents' struggle to reconsummate their joining despite overwhelming odds points to the transformational passion of the sacred union of male and female. The welcome my grandfather extends to my mother and me so honors the maternal feminine that his greeting feels like a joyous reunion after a long and painful absence, or the fulfillment of reconciliation with one who has been lost.

As he greets us with love, he calls my mother "Nana," which is one of the names of Inanna, Sumerian goddess of the upper world, original mother of all. To regain wholeness, Inanna descends into her sister's domain in the agony of the underworld. It is a necessary journey into her shadowed depths to reclaim lost pieces of herself. In that descent, Inanna is reborn. She remembers who she is.

This dream brings together archetypal images of the feminine, the Three in One: mother, maiden, and crone. In it, my mother is a guide to my ancient roots, to the home of my ancestors. Rather than instructed or directed,

I feel deeply companioned by she who matters: my mother. She grounds me in the ways of the earth and represents the quality of feminine companionship and nurturing.

The daughter–maiden aspect of my dream and my psyche represents life's endless regeneration. She is soul—the eternal vitality of hope and expectancy contained within her self, assurance within the maternal.

Mother and maiden grow and mature with the wise crone's imprint embedded in their becoming. This old woman knows the earth's rhythms and has seen life begin and end again. Chronic illness has forced me into a level of inner crone work prematurely. Sometimes I feel it is work better suited to the very old.

In this dream, my grandmother-crone is girlishly delighted with herself, as if she keeps a wonderful secret. She is bald. No outer manifestation of achievement, performance, or even beauty has anything at all to do with her inner qualities. She is enough just as she is, and she knows it.

Her beloved, my grandfather, honors the nature of the feminine and is not there to tell any of the women in my dream what to do. He beholds us in love: with fatherly devotion for my mother aspect, grandfatherly protection for my inner maiden, and sacred desire for my grandmother-crone.

I see this as indicating my old attitudes must die as I grow into the experience of who I am—maiden, mother, and crone—in my life as it now is. Rigid definitions of normalcy must give way to more flexible attitudes toward my life. I am learning that spiritual growth is possible in the painstaking work of bringing the opposites together.

The life–death–life archetype appears in my dream as that suffering and death offer me a vision of new life: of healing into wholeness far beyond my greatest anticipation. Nowhere is that more passionate than in the *conjunctio* of man and woman, the original prototype of opposites. The dream signifies that the relationship of masculine and feminine in my psyche is becoming one of mutuality rather than patriarchy.

When we consciously carry the suffering of unresolved polarities (illness and health, for example), the realness of both extremes becomes clear. Opposites usually fight to win out over each other, yet when I choose to hold this tension in balance neither can consume me. In their mutuality and splendor, the opposites of male and female are like two pieces of wood, smoothed and polished to reveal the beauty of their inner grains. In joining, they can touch on every surface and part freely to move and attend to their own individuation. In such sacred joining without snarls and entanglements, wholeness is incarnate in the world and God is born again. "When opposites touch," says Albert Kreinheder,* "a tremendous energy is released. Miracles of healing

---

Body and Soul, p. 27.

are then possible and astonishing disturbances, both good and bad, occur."

No longer shuffling in dreamlight, my grandfather is now a guide who helps me measure the steps on my path of individuation and connects me to my destiny.

> For each child that's born,
> A morning star rises
> And sings to the universe who we are.
> We are our grandmother's prayers.
> We are our grandfather's dreamings.
> We are the breath of our ancestors.
> We are the spirit of God.
>
> *—of Yiddish origin*

GRANNY

Granny is dead. Cold, unwanted syllables tumble around my tongue in strange and unfamiliar ways. I've never put these three words together before. They are hollow and unreal to my ears.

Granny had eaten breakfast and then rolled her long, thin gray hair around her two hair rats, which perched on either side of her head. Long U-shaped hairpins pulled up the hair above her face and held it in a biscuit. For as long as I can recall, she had saved each strand of hair that fell out into her brush and wound it mindfully around

103

and around the rat. I never tired of gazing at my grand-mother repeat her oblations in just the same way each morning.

That particular morning, the morning she died, was no different. She smoothed rose water and glycerin into her skin until she fairly glistened with moisture. Her hair up and a dab of lipstick rubbed into her cheeks, a little powder on her nose, and she was ready for my mother to help her into her corset and dress. Oh, that corset! I watched in amazement as Granny pushed and pulled her flesh into the corset form, held tight by long plastic stays, hooks, and laces. She then settled into her chair with an unmistakable air of genuine friendly refinement, her eyes sparkling as if to say, "I have a secret." She was ready to preside for the day.

An unexpected silence settled around my mother and grandmother. Their morning conversation over Postum was left hanging in mid air. Granny heaved a great sigh, bowed her head, and died. Right there like that.

Like that. That's the way a Southern lady wants to die, I had heard. My father's mother had died that way, too. Dressed for the day and presiding from her chair, Grandma Lessie had said, "I feel sooooo tired." Tilted her head to one side and was gone.

Granny chose to be cremated. It seems an unlikely choice for an elderly Southern woman thirty years ago.

I've often wondered if my father talked her into it. Then again, Granny was always open to different ideas. Nothing that I ever told her seemed to shock her.

She would have loved our gathering in the basement after her memorial service. My parents, my mother's brother Marvin, my sisters Priscilla and Katharine, and I gathered to open Granny's trunk. Even my mother had never opened Granny's trunk. My heart was about to jump out of my skin. I felt as if we were going to look upon the face of God.

Dried and cracking leather straps came together at the rusty metal lock of the old brown wooden trunk. With a few efforts in assisting key and lock, my mother opened it. A puff of mothball scent welcomed us into family mysteries of days and months and years gone by. We found letters, Granny's school slate, and photographs and sketches my grandfather had made of the Lumbee Indians, a tribe indigenous to the part of North Carolina where she lived.

Of all the treasures we found that day, the most wondrous was Granny's brown silk shantung wedding suit, her high-heeled button shoes, and a hat with poofed veiling now limp with age which at one time must have looked very sassy. Folded in tissue paper under all that was her honeymoon's white satin nightgown, now yellowed.

What happened next seemed like sheer magic. With scarcely any hesitation, my mother stepped out of her own dress and slipped into Granny's suit and shoes. They fit perfectly. Leaping into the center of his own excitement, my father needed only gentle urging to retrieve his squeezebox accordion from upstairs. While he played, my mother danced and danced and danced. "See us now, Granny. This is for you!" We laughed and cried and loved Granny and each other with our whole hearts.

So it is that my days connect with my mother's days and Granny's days as well, for we are indivisibly connected though destined to suffer our own sufferings.

REALITIES

After my diagnosis, I automatically shifted into living my life in two realities: the reality of figuring out the practical, day-in-day-out problems and challenges of maintaining my quality of life; and an inner spiritual reality concerned with meanings and soulful questions. Who am I now, and who am I becoming? This spiritual reality both permeates and transcends my mundane reality.

My practical reality is scrupulously attentive to the details of scheduling and preparing medications, noting changes in my symptoms, planning events around the times when I expect to be most flexible. This includes making plane reservations for when I expect to be "on," or moving normally; or scheduling dinner to follow my last medication for the day, when I can eat protein. (Protein greatly inhibits the effectiveness of one of my medications, Sinemet.)

Most importantly, my day-to-day reality focuses on maintaining ready supplies of medications and my pharmacological equipment for making liquid Sinemet each day, as it is unavailable on the market in this form. As my need for Sinemet varies with changes in my metabolism, activity level, and stress, having it in liquid form gives me more control over how often and how much I ingest.

I take my portable apothecary with me everywhere. It is not unlike the basket of a tribal medicine woman with her paraphernalia of rattles and feathers, herbs and potions. Both of us practice protection through ritual. My medicine bag is a bright purple, insulated picnic container with two zippered compartments. These hold my three medications (Sinemet, Eldepryl, and Permax), ascorbic acid, mortar and pestle, graduated cylinder, spoons, plastic bottles of various sizes, bottle brushes, funnels, vitamins, nutrition supplements, herbal remedies, teas, flavored drink mix, dried fruit, and water. Very often, I include an object of healing power—such as a special rock, an artifact, or crystal—that at the time carries recuperative properties for me. Finally are my journal and pens for recording experiences of meaning.

This array of allopathic medicines and complementary treatment supplements bewilders any onlooker when I make my brew. Once, wearily awaiting my final flight after a long day's travel, I had to laugh when I thought about how I might look to fellow passengers in the waiting area as I set up my portable apothecary on a borrowed suitcase. I had run out of my premixed medication and had to prepare a new batch quickly. In just minutes, my body would use up the Sinemet I had taken earlier.

If I skip or postpone medication, my vitality and flexibility drop suddenly. Muscles tighten and I move more and more slowly. Fear and helplessness crowd out optimism and well being. When this happens—and it does happen—I focus full attention on breathing in and breathing out to stay calm. Then I reach with all my heart for spirit: for the strength and hope that is greater than I.

Within that greater reality nestle the soul, depth, and mystery of my being. There, an attentive quality of life is responsive to meaningfulness, matters of the heart, and the experience of things eternal. This reality gives my heart strength and direction. It brings spiritual meaning to day-to-day specifics by patterning life-force energy to truths and themes from the wisdom reservoir of all humankind. This is the realm of archetypal healing through dreams and symbols, visions and synchronicities, story and metaphor, art, poetry—in short, through the imaginal. Accepting life with all of its horrors and in all of its beauty in the inner connectedness of all that is brings me to God.

One encounter that points to a deeper, broader patterning in my life, an awakening to the sacred, occurred while I was dining out with friends on an island in the Caribbean Sea. Absorbed in the succulence of local lobster and grilled bananas, I suddenly felt gentle hands touching my shoulders. My body softened instantly into what felt like a healer's touch. Turning my head, I saw our server, a regal black woman, perhaps in her mid-thirties, bending over me, our faces only inches apart. In her Caribbean accent, which to me sounded more like song than speech, she asked, "What is your name?"

"Lessie Anne," I replied, giving her my full name instead of the shortened version, Les, which most people call me.

Three times she spoke it—"Lessie Anne, Lessie Anne, Lessie Anne"—with care and sweetness that moved me deeply. I asked her name. "Feronica," she replied.

Looking into her dark and compassionate face, I followed suit. "Feronica, Feronica, Feronica." Tears came to my eyes, and I am certain I saw them in hers.

The moment passed. For a while, no one at our table spoke. All recognized the occurrence of something profound.

Later, as we paddled our dinghy back out to our moored sailboat, I saw Feronica waving goodbye from the pier. At four o'clock in the morning, I awoke weeping tears of deep feeling. In my sorrow, I had received comfort from a stranger far from my home. Somehow, we knew one another's hearts and felt the kinship of sisters without any stories. What transpired is not comprehensible through rationality, yet its effect on me continues.

Feronica became for me a beautiful image representing a great truth about the depth and alighting of love: that compassion stems from grace, and that love may come to warm our lives as if on the wings of an angel. This is the dimension of mystery, of meaningfulness, in which our ordinary interactions reveal a deeper level of purposeful design. In my spiritual journeying, this experience came at a time when I longed for the comfort of feminine consolation.

HEALING STORIES
AND RITUALS

On hot summer nights, my family often piled into our 1965 Chevy stationwagon and headed for the shores of Lake Texoma, eager for the breeze that rippled across the water. On the cool, moist sand, parents and young ones alike would stretch out in a circle, our heads meeting with whispers at the center. As we drew in the sand and listened to the waves lapping lazily at the water's edge, hours passed in the dark of night and babies eased into sleep.

The big Texas sky extended endlessly, its silver-white moon and galaxies of stars infinitely remote, awesome in their splendor, and insistent in nudging us to share the stories they stirred in us. These stories told of the great unknowns and incomprehensibilities, and of the mysteries of life, death, and all dimensions between. Our tales reached for the infinite and for the wisdom of life.

Decades later, I still need my stories, my dreams, my mythologies, my rituals. As eternity breaks into time through ritual and story, their enduring truths and ageless motifs connect me to the circle of all life. Like dreams, stories and ritual are plump with archetypal potential. Their themes and ideas grip us as we travel the boundaries between known and unknown, searching for a recognizable world in the formlessness of life's calamities.

Stories and rituals awaken us to consciousness and sometimes to the healing of heartache and depression. Stories of creation call us into life—to the dawning of our existence—and help us comprehend the mysteries of our yearnings and ambivalence, our urgencies and commonalties, our defeats and sorrowing. In the calling, telling, and performance, we recognize a significant and meaningful, even patterned world inherent in the chaotic darkness of our lives. For me, stories and rituals prevent my fate of Parkinson's from victimizing me, for they transform my fate into meaningful experience.

I need to bring purpose and form to the themes and patterns of this life I live—to write and draw, dance and sing my personal fate. In the mystery of illness, words and silences speak of the body–mind and express the soul. Through its constraints, Parkinson's apparent limiting story invites me to live into a larger, deeper story in which synchronicities link people and phenomena in experience rich with meaning and intent. Nothing is irrelevant in that tale, in which all that is and has been comes together in one place, like the place in the acorn that imagines the tree.

Dreams, stories, and rituals also mirror us—expose us for who we are and are not—and provide images whose power may transform us. Jamake Highwater's book *Anpao* is a composite story from generations of

Great Plains and Southwest native peoples. It includes a beautiful creation story of how Old Man, the allspirit, created the world and its inhabitants. Here is a paraphrase of my favorite part:

> After creating the sea creatures that live on the surface of water, such as geese and mallards, loons and coots, Old Man gave them freedom also to fly. What a joyous celebration that was, with all varieties of birds splashing and skimming the surface of lakes and rivers. Old Man created a beautiful sky in which the birds could also soar.
>
> But between swimming and flying, there was no soil on which they might land and rest. As Old Man had already created much and was tired, he asked the creatures of the air for help.

To create land would be an immense task, so the birds exclaimed, "We must *find* land!" The swiftest and strongest of them flapped their powerful wings and flew into the sky, nearly out of sight, turned, "and plummeting down like an arrow, dived into the water to look for land." One brave goose was under water a very long time but returned with nothing.

While this was happening, Little Coot, the smallest of the sea creatures, had been dipping his head in and out of the water, chirping happily as he paddled about. When the goose returned with nothing, Little Coot offered his service to Old Man. "Old Man," Little Coot whispered, "when I dip my head into the green water, I think I see something there—very, very far below, in the dark. I am small, I know, but perhaps I can swim deep enough to reach it. I cannot fly high into the sky, nor can I dive like my brothers and sisters. I can only swim. But I will try my best to swim deep into the water and find what we are looking for."

"Try, little brother," said Old Man.

"Ah-ho!" the little coot replied. He tipped his head under water and was gone, down and down into the water. He dove to where it was the greenest, which meant it was the deepest.

Little Coot was underwater for a very long time—so long that Old Man worried that some harm had come to him. Finally, he saw a very small dark spot in the water. The spot rose and rose until Old Man and the sea creatures could see Little Coot struggling to reach the water's surface.

"What have you brought?" Old Man asked as he held his hand under the coot's beak. A small ball of mud fell into his hand.

Old Man was very pleased. As he rolled the mud in his hands, it grew and grew until he could not hold it any longer. He looked about to find Grandmother Turtle, who would carry the pile of mud on her back. And Earth was created.

This story joins the powerful, androgynous omnipresence of Old Man with his shadow aspect, the coot. This smallest of the birds, with childlike devotion and instinctive knowing, accomplishes what the larger creatures cannot. Rather than straining to push beyond his natural means, Little Coot gracefully tips under water and swims deep. He willingly risks everything to do what he does naturally with innate skill. He does what's *true*. That is exactly what is needed, as is the give-back of Grandmother Turtle. For her patience and strength of age, Old Man chooses her to carry land on her back.

Listening to his inner voice, Little Coot trusts himself to unknown depths. That voice sends no messages of inferiority or greedy ambition to diminish his unique and authentic contribution. He gives of who he is naturally. Knowing his own nature, he finds a way to serve with congruence. Even a tiny ball of mud can be precisely what is needed.

So it is for each of us as we seek expression for our own offerings. It is the heart's intent rather than the gift's size that matters most. Wounded and ill, we may require care; but when we tell our stories, we are caring for others through the truth of our words. Even afflictions may become a source of power in our gifts and strength in our spirits as we make our contribution.

Touching not only our intellect but also that which is immortal, stories that honor the creator open depths of unconscious wisdom in each of us. They make sense of the senseless. They point to life as a passionate force in which transformative powers are evoked. Many traditional peoples believe that chanting creation stories for seven sacred days and nights over the body of an ill person invites and mobilizes healing energies implicit in the process of creation itself.

As parables do, such rituals around stories create a vessel to hold the power of images—a space to receive and incubate healing archetypal energy. They may be complex events such as fasting and participating in rounds of the sweat lodge, or simple personal actions and gestures of spirit that acknowledge the sacred power to which we surrender. Struggling with her own condition,lupus, Laura Chester writes tenderly:*

> I found myself wanting to open my hands in the gesture of receiving, my head lifted rather than bowed. I still felt humble and small, yet glad in this upwardness, imagining light pouring into me, healing me, gathering me up and holding

---

* *Lupus Novice, p. 79.*

me . . .. I could feel the need to bare the smallest part of myself, the tiny seed self, to expose
what was essentially me, pitiful, painful, vulnerable, to hold that out, as if to shining rain.

The creative use of stories and rituals involves gathering life-force energy for healing and guidance. Without
a conscious decision, I have discovered abiding comfort
in my own nightly ritual of singing hymns and spontaneous chanting. No longer do I dread lying awake in the
middle of the night with or without dystonia or other
discomforts. I know the mystery of the night well; it is
also part of the gold I mine. I sing hymns quietly beside
J. Linn, or I make up new songs so that my attention is
absorbed in creative activity. My feet may be cramping

terribly, yet I am aware of the cramping more as sensation, not so much as pain. Something more engaging than physical discomfort occupies my mind. The simple ritual of singing hymns I learned as a child releases my suffering in the night. The compelling desire to sing creates a trance of heightened awareness that makes pain bearable. At other times, I must bear the misery.

On occasion, I discover depth and meaning when I join with others to call in the four directions, in the Native American way. With the sound of the drum drawing us to sacred space, I yield to the heartbeat of Earth as she gathers me unto herself. Tears of homecoming moisten and soften my body's aches and tight places, which are the consequences I now face to keep moving.

As we fan the sacred smoke that encircles us and carries our prayers heavenward, I raise my arms in praise and surrender. Turning to honor and welcome the spirits of the east, south, west, and north with invocations and singing, I offer myself to God, to the Great Spirit, to the Goddess of the Deep for healing. Rituals and stories lift me from the prison of Parkinson's limitations and burdens.

From the simple offering of Little Coot grew the vast and powerful earth, whose warm and loamy darkness embraced Old Man when it came time for him to breathe his last. As he dropped his knees onto the rich soil of the earth, which he had created, form began to emerge from within, even in death. The great waters flowed from his mouth while the light of dawn made love with the colors of the setting sun. Life's rapture became complete.

DESCENT AND ASCENT
OF THE DEEP FEMININE

Stories sing the miracle of creation into words as soil vibrates life into seeds. Joined with Earth—her dark, moist essence my own affiliation—I become a vessel for receiving and caressing the seeds and bulbs of new life. They burrow and nestle into my soul-flesh like the words of stories that press into my psyche, growing tendrils to increase with strength as they wind their rootlets around me and through me, over and under me. They create an intricate web of reciprocity that presses downward into the world beneath the world.

Stories lure us into mysterious depths, into regions of instinct and imagination. They take us even into dis-integration, where the forces of being try to overwhelm the hardy ego, where underground waters bathe fossils and bones—the present inhabitants of the great below—and shadows cast ominous images upon the path that leads deep and down. This is a_story of downgoings. This is also the story of the feminine rising from her ancient roots to sacred awakenings.

Great stories or myths parallel our seemingly cha-otic and mundane lives. They illuminate and even heal our personal suffering and brokenness. Thus, I find my encounter with Parkinson's mirrored in the ancient story of Inanna and Ereshkigal. This is a story of the descent of the feminine into her depths to confront a dark and wounded side of herself, and in the rawness of that encounter, Inanna brings forth a more whole feminine.

My life before Parkinson's is much like Inanna's, a story of pushing and searching for success in the outer world. Then, like she, I was called into the depths to confront Ereshkigal, in the form of Parkinson's. This illness is transforming my life from being driven to being receptive, from a patriarchal need for control to feminine understanding, from getting the job done no matter what to regarding each person and event as unique.

Hear first my personal story of over-striving for success and then the ancient story from Mesopotamia. Born in Wilmington, North Carolina, I spent my growing-up years in Louisville, Kentucky and began school at Longfellow Elementary. Enthusiasm for this new venture, which my mother fostered, lasted less than an hour. I made an awful discovery that first day.

Unless we were sight- or hearing-impaired, we sat in rows, our desks bolted to the floor. Since my last name begins with the letter *R*, my assigned desk was at the back of the room. This was a shock. I wanted to be in the front, close tothe teacher. Said to be the best teacher in the whole school, she incessantly patted the heads of her front-row students, calling them by name and affectionately designating them her "little cabbage heads." I would never get to be a cabbage head! That was quite clear. And I hated those who did.

Teachers early in our lives are so important to us. They are, in fact, surrogate mothers, and we are their children. If I could not be a cabbage head, I surmised, my teacher didn't love me.

Second grade was tedious, and I often found myself in trouble for talking with my neighbors. Our third-grade class was so large that three of us girls skipped third grade. I think my two friends and I were chosen because we were already buddies, and I was tall. We landed in the fourth-grade class, where neither teacher nor students wanted us. The teacher told us not to expect special treatment for being younger than our classmates.

She did assign us desks in the front of the room, thinking we'd pay better attention there. My seat was directly in front of her desk, which sat on a platform raised about a foot above the floor. My forward gaze was right into Miss Beeler's crotch! I spent my whole year trying to avert my eyes from her pink flared under-drawers.

I laugh about this now. The serious aspect, though, is that my drive to strive began as a compensation for feeling inadequate behind and trying to catch up. I learned to push on, hiding my fears and desires to belong while pretending not to care. Feeling behind and ashamed of being behind, feeling inadequate yet determined to catch up no matter what—these have haunted me much of my life.

Another factor in my drive for success has to do with my love and care for Virginia Satir. The world was Virginia's home and, as an extrovert, she seemed to thrive on a life of public visibility. She nudged me to put my name in neon lights. That also appealed to me. At last I would become a cabbage head. Yet, as an introvert, for me with my life story, that was not authentic ambition.

From 1974 to 1984, I was living out an intense decade of immense drive. It included returning to graduate school for a degree in counseling, a move from Illinois to North Carolina, separation, divorce, and being a single mom with two children. My professional energies went to teaching part time at Duke University, building a psychotherapy practice, and presenting workshops and lectures. My feminine authority had been captivated by an inflated focus on achievement thatseparated me from my authentic nature.

Six years into this pattern of overdrive, an unexpected and amazing thing occurred. I was enraptured by love for a dear friend of twenty years. J. Linn and I married in 1986. The joy of our coming together after years of friendship released a source of energy that poured forth like a geyser. No challenge was too formidable. With that abundance, I had to *do* something in the world. It never occurred to me to use this vitality to savor *being* in the world.

In addition to building a psychotherapy practice near my new home in the mountains, I commuted back to the North Carolina Triangle three days a week to see clients there. I also taught part time at Appalachian State University. Even this was not enough, so I began a doctoral program with Union Institute.

Mobilizing so much energy for the world's acknowledgment meant living in the future, preoccupied with plans and goals. What I missed in my drive to excel, my addiction to achievement, was the preciousness of life's ordinary moments. Not long after, I felt the first symptoms of Parkinson's.

It has taken chronic illness to bend me low enough to get the lessons. Instead of hard drive, I now surrender to the tempo of nature. I am learning to sit on the earth to *receive* my life, morning by morning, as the night becomes dawn and the dark becomes light. At the boundary between the two is the eternal moment, the still point, a reverent pause that celebrates the birth of a new day. The regularity of nature's patterns comforts me during this intense time.

This condition presents me with a recurring cycle of wretched descents and ascents to remind me of the lessons. At times, my body's search for dopamine forces me to descend into ugly and hidden spaces of Earth's wilderness that torment my flesh and batter my spirit. The worst of my descent comes at the crossroads. There I may hang ten minutes or two hours, trapped between the agonizing struggle of being neither "on" nor "off" my medication, but liminal, trapped between polarities, my muscles and nerve endings scrambled and chaotic. Some of my muscles seem to shut down while others fight for their lives, prodding me to keep moving. From bed to chair to floor, I push and coax my body on. Stifled cries of illness become whimpers of staggering grief as I crawl on hands and knees in my effort to keep moving.

Here I am defenseless, stripped of all resources. I plead for God to help me. Hubris absolved, humility assured. Desperate and afraid, overwhelmed and worn down, I cry out for the love of God. I am surprised that lyrics from music performed years ago appear spontaneously in memory.

Oh, turn me not away.
Hear thou my cry.
Hear thou my cry.
Oh Lord hear my distress
And hasten to my aid.*

Words I learned at the knee of patriarchy serve me until I feel stripped down to nothing. I am in the vise of Parkinson's and forced to surrender. "You win." Then something seems to happen. I let go of hubris, conceit, and desires. I accept what feels like the loss of everything. There is then a change. A transformation begins. Reaching my lowest ebb, I feel an eternal presence touching me with kindness—a feminine consciousness that comes to bless

---

*"O Divine Redeemer," aria by Gonoud.

me and inform me that I am strengthened and toughened by the ordeal. I have endured and discover that the dark instinct of my nature has reclaimed me. The goddess of earth who was with me in my dream of the irises is with me now. With poignancy and understanding, Clarissa Estes* describes these dark times, when

> the feminine unconscious, the uterine unconscious, Nature, feeds a woman's soul. . . . in the midst of their descent they are in the darkest dark and are touched by the brush of a wing tip and feel light-ened. They feel an inner nourishing taking place, a spring of blessed water bursting forth over parched ground . . .This spring does not solve suffering,

---

Women Who Run with the Wolves, p. 415.

but rather nourishes when nothing else is forth-
coming. It is manna in the desert. It is water from
stones. It is food out of thin air. It quells the hunger
so we can go on. And that is the whole point . . . to
go on. To go on toward our knowing destiny.

As quickly as immobility descends on me, it now
lifts and I am restored to normal movement, free of pain,
a song in my heart. *The strife is ore the battle done. The
victory of life is won. The song of triumph has begun.
Alleluia!* Thus, I discover that for every descent in this
cycle, there is a return; for every ascent, a down-going.
One round of descent reveals another in this ritual of

---

*"The Strife Is O'er," *The Presbyterian Hymnal* (1990), p. 119.

endurance. The way down is perilous for me and yet calls to me with an allurement to know and understand the ingredients and the lessons of my sorrow and suffering as well as the qualities required to integrate my illness and regain my strength. I reclaim parts of myself which I now need for wholeness, especially my lust for life, my vitality of spirit, my capacity to cry out and summon forth my courage and my wildness: the cry and whisper of my true nature.

From 6,000 years before Christ, the following ancient ritual and story call to me and connect to my own life story of over-striving in the outer world and to my Parkinson's cycle of descending and ascending. In her book *Uncursing the Dark,* Betty Meador, a Jungian analyst, has researched and written about the time and the rite of Thesmophoria. This ancient Sumerian ritual acknowledged the power and mystery of women to grow the crops with the flesh and blood of their menses.

Even without words, I sense a deep and primal pull into a dark abyss where the repressed powers of women await retrieving from a distant time. With those of us who honor the full capacity of feminine emotion, passion and the numinous compel us to receive the deep feminine. As women and men today, we find ancient and primal stories that bear on our psyches and origins.

To prepare for three days of the Thesmophoria, women intentionally withdrew from community life in ancient times, writes Meador. * In those days, it was customary for women to make a descent literally, carrying fat piglets down into a lair of snakes. They believed snakes to be holy carriers of life within Earth. There, they sacrificed the pigs to honor Snake, to express the earth's holiness, to name the great powers of being around which they oriented their lives, and to remind them that, through the earth, Snake's power was available to them.

Aligning with the merciless detachment of Snake, the women told and enacted stories with searing honesty

---

* *Uncursing the Dark,* p. 64.

about what they saw of one another in day-to-day village life. Meador describes this:*

> Passion stirs and rises. They begin to shout at each other. What has been tolerated, ignored, hidden, is exposed. They hurl scurrilous remarks, scathing, burning descriptions that image details of acts of utmost privacy . . .. They rage. They cry. They fight, hurl clods and stones. No one is spared. Secrets, hatreds, envies, jealousies are all exposed. A woman cannot avoid seeing her secret self made public. . . . The shouting exposes secrets, shatters pride, levels the women to common ground. . . . The women are mortified. They are stripped of pride, foolish desire. . . . Snake's gifts of sight and fecundity are only a thin line

---

*Uncursing the Dark, pp. 98–99.

removed from her [the woman's] powers of wild posses-
sion and madness.

After deep sleep, the women completed the Thesmophoria by taking pig flesh and seed corn from the altar
to the fields. As they pressed seed and flesh into the
earth, they lifted their voices to sing the praises of Snake,
whom they called Ereshkigal.

Ereshkigal: symbol of the unconscious, the instinctual feminine. Queen of the dark pit, fecund and un-
kempt, impersonal and vengeful, demanding a sacrifice
of no less than all the sociocultural achievements a
woman had attained. Ereshkigal: whose heart softens
to allow transformation in a woman's life. Ereshkigal:

who presides over the terror and suffering of death and the struggle for breath in new life.

I first met this goddess on my forty-third birthday, when my sister gave me a copy of Sylvia Brinton Perera's book *Descent to the Goddess: A Way of Initiation for Women.* That was a time just after divorce, relocation, and new professional directions had plunged me into my own descent. Perera's book validated the process of change that I was experiencing. It sustained my conviction to keep moving even in times of weakness, fear, and self-doubt. It confirmed my reaching for the support of other women and the earth's warmth, and it honored an image from my unconscious of a deep and strong-flowing underground river that knows its course seaward.

Perera's book also introduced me to the story from 3,500 B.C. of Inanna, queen of the upper world, and Ereshkigal, goddess of the netherworld. Again and again over the ensuing years, I have returned to this myth for feminine renewal. Especially now, as I seek to give birth to myself in a journey of spiritual descent which must necessarily include the labyrinth of chronic disablement, I find guidance and solace in this story, which I summarize here.

> Wearing the royal finery of her seven garments of power, Inanna, queen of the upper world, descends into her sister Ereshkigal's pit of darkness. Through her suffering, we will see how Inanna releases her condescending ways to find the natural realness of her deep feminine self, that eternal patterning which gives meaning to her life.

151

Ereshkigal is furious that Inanna has dared come to her realm. Consumed by envy, she instructs her judges to strip Inanna of her finery and any remnant of superiority as she proceeds through the seven entry gates.

At the first gate, they take away Inanna's headdress, symbol of intellectual development and illumination in the upper world. At each succeeding gate, they divest her regal masks, jewelry, awards, and accoutrements. Ultimately, she stands naked and humiliated, all arrogance gone, before the dark goddess, her sister Ereshkigal.

Inanna and Ereshkigal point to the light and dark sides of each other. Although they are two aspects of one woman, in this story they are estranged, body split from soul, spirit cut off from body. In *Like Gold Through*

Fire (p. 55), Massimilla and Bud Harris emphasize the pain that results from such a rupture:

> Ereshkigal represents the neglected side of Inanna, including her instinctive, compulsive, insatiable, and sexual characteristics. Ereshkigal also includes the wounded and frightened parts of Inanna, the parts Inanna had rejected from her conscious identity, stripping them of respect and reverence and a place in her life. It's not surprising that, in these circumstances, these denied parts might become an adversary whose aim is to kill and destroy.

Indeed, Ereshkigal's disowned aspects do become vicious. In her fury and anguish, Ereshkigal decrees that Inanna be hung on a peg like a piece of rotting meat until she dies. Like Inanna, those of us challenged by

153

chronic health situations—physical or mental—may experience the loss of independence and dignity as a vicious stripping away of identity. Without mercy and with similar vengeance, illness shoves us into a descent toward the threshold of life and death, where physical suffering and incapacitation remind us of Inanna's fate and Ereshkigal's woundedness. Piece by piece, one accomplishment after another, Inanna loses her identity until nothing of her fame and stardom remains.

Linked to universal stories that animate life, our personal stories become more bearable. Those of us who see Inanna's suffering and Ereshkigal's indignation as our own may find that tale offers direction for finding safe ways to express emotions suppressed into containment within our bodies' cells. And if we see the seven gates as corresponding to the seven *chakras,* or energy centers of the body, we may understand that Inanna's divestiture—her release from cultural expectations—opens her for transformation. Change is stirring in both sisters as the paraphrase continues.

> While Inanna suffers and dies, we learn that Ereshkigal is pregnant and in hard labor, groaning and moaning with pain as she prepares to bring forth new life. Death leading not to death but to life.
>
> Having slipped in unnoticed by the guards at the gates, two very small mourners place themselves beside Ereshkigal to commiserate: "Poor Ereshkigal. Such hard work this labor is! Ah, your insides hurt. And your outsides, too. Ooooh. Ahhhh. Ooooh. Poor, dear Ereshkigal."

155

> Their sincere compassion so moves Ereshkigal that her heart softens. Unexpectedly, she grants Inanna's return to life in the upper world. On the third day, Inanna rises from the dead.

This reminds us of grief's potential for new life. In the darkness of our deepest losses, grief's gold awaits our undertaking to mine it.

Inanna and Ereshkigal cover their deep vulnerabilities with defensive stances. Inanna's arrogance is a cover for fear and the longing for love. Ereshkigal's fury masks her dependence, shame, and her need of love. Each desperately seeks the other for her wholeness. Their defensiveness is mobilized to cope with the pain of splitting body from soul Were we to peel away that which is present but unspoken, I believe we might hear a revealing exchange.

"How dare you appear unannounced in my domain?" Ereshkigal might protest. "What audacity! Have you come from your high and mighty throne in the upper world to judge me? To stand so arrogantly above me in your finery? To gawk at my miserable misfortune? Do you want to thank the gods that you've escaped my fate?

"You were always a know-it-all, Inanna. You think you're better than the rest of us. What can you know of real suffering? My suffering doesn't stop. I'm despised and rejected, flawed, crippled, unwanted, and humiliated. I can hardly bear myself!

"But I don't want your pity. I don't even want you to look at me. I remember the upper world only too well, with all its standards of perfection: look immaculate, stylish, pretty—unencumbered by any weakness, flaws, or disability. And if you do have the misfortune of disfigurement, at least try to *look* normal. What matters is appearance. Don't deviate from the standard. Be who the powerful ones think you should be. Look good whether you feel good or not. Don't be who you really are. Don't say what you really think. You'll only look stupid. It's the show that matters.

"Look! Yes, *do* look at me. What you see is who I am. Look closely, Inanna, because what you see is who *you* are, too. You and I are forever indivisible. I am part of you, and you're part of me. Like it or not, that's the way it is.

"Your arrival is a torture, for my wretchedness shows more clearly in the light you've brought with you. Go. Go away! Too much light—you'll blind me.

"No, stay. I lie. I'm only a fragile creature hiding out in my rage and fear. I'm ashamed for you to see me as I am now. I hate my state. I hate it! I despise my dependence and my weakness. How to bear my lot?

"How to bear the heaviness of my sadness? That's the challenge. A lesson in losses, that is my life! My grief, a daily mourning. I am one who grieves her inescapable sorrow. Is it even possible for one so fragile as I to be loved?"

159

Inanna might respond, "What you say about me is true, Ereshkigal. I am judgmental. I am haughty. And I am condescending. But please believe me, I'm not here to pour salt in your wounds. I've risked no less than everything I have gained to come before you.

"You have something I do not: you know deeply about life and death. That's the reason I am here. You have a relationship with life's dark side. And I long for that—for my dark sister. I cannot be whole without you.

"Yes, I am prideful and competitive, independent and cold. I have pleased the powerful ones. I am a warrior woman and can show off well in the upper world, but I am restless, without peace.

"My sadness is so profound as to touch a fragile and needy child who lives in my musings. She is so alone. I have no home, no place to call mine. No soul to console the tears of my sorrowing. The reed does not know how to bend.

"This is what lies behind my driven state, my love of fame, my addiction to achievement. I dare not stop, lest my life collapse. I am a fake, Ereshkigal. My fine robes cover my emptiness and my endless sadness. I am lost, Ereshkigal! What is to become of me?"

"Inanna must go down," writes Perera,

> to meet her own instinctual beginnings. Inanna must go down into the depths of her feelings, into her terror, lostness and sorrowing to find

161

the face of the Great Goddess and of herself
before she was born to consciousness.*

It is to heal the break between opposites in her life—the
light and the dark, body and spirit—that Inanna must
descend into her sister's netherworld. The refined and
successful persona she shows to the world must join
with the unacceptable, shameful, hate-filled aspects of
her hidden self. It is separation that estranges us from
ourselves and each other. From that brutal split in
ourselves come the atrocities that any person inflicts on
another, any nation on another. Inanna must go down
into the mine to learn that she and Ereshkigal are one.

---

*Descent to the Goddess, p. 45.

To find the whole of who I am, likewise, requires peeling back my successful exterior and inching down into my own shadowy parts: my fears, grief, and feeling of loss. Beyond the struggle between overdrive and inertia, I am now exploring a third response to living: one of process, feminine consciousness rooted in a practical vision and belief in reality unseen. A response that values flow and adaptation, that reveals the wisdom of quietude and calm, that supports diving into my darkest depths to bring up the power of life's renewal, that supports my life's force to express the way of the wild. My heart softens to receive the gift of being loved, even in my deepest shame and darkest despair. That is gold mined from the dark of the great below.

Stories reveal the abiding presence of the archetypal, the universal feminine in our lives. As I am willing to see your suffering and reveal mine to you, we become one. Being reborn spiritually entails our descent into Earth's labyrinth, where we discover that the deep feminine has been present all our lives.

Even in childhood, we may have heard the voice of a deep feminine authority speaking through us. I remember an occasion of such conscious identification at age seven. My father had chosen me to go with him to the grocery store. This was a special event, as he was not home often during his days as a seminary scholar and minister. Dancing with glee and anticipation, I hurried to unlatch the side door to the car. I wanted to please him with my helpfulness, but the lock jammed.

"Darn, darn, *DARN!*" Flaring, I stammered the most mature response I could think of at that moment.

"No daughter of mine will use that kind of language!" my father rebuked me. "And if she does, she won't be going to the store—or anywhere else, for that matter." I was shocked and devastated. There must be some mistake. My mother said "darn" a lot.

He rebuffed my apology and sent me to my room as I begged him not to leave me behind. Then he rebuked me for my tears: "And if you don't stop crying, I'll give you something to cry about."

In that moment, a surge of awareness shook me to my foundation. Simultaneously, I heard a voice resounding from my body and beyond: "NO!" "You may *never* take my tears away. They're *mine*. My tears! Besides, I can't make my tears go away. That's the way tears are." Then and there as I climbed the stairs to my room, I vowed that when I became a parent, I would never try to stop my child's tears.

Later, in the evening after my outburst, the surprising gentleness in my father's voice touched my heart. He had heard and respected me. Even at seven, owning my tears came from a place of deep authority, the power of deep feminine instinct, the power of Ereshkigal and Inanna. Many years later, I understood his fear of my childhood emotions: they mirrored his own unshed tears.

Though young, my instinctual self found the integrity and confidence to meet patriarchy head on, to speak with energetic faithfulness to my nature and my truth, as I believed it to be. I loved myself fiercely in that moment. That experience has reverberated in my life every day since with a love for all who struggle to give voice to their truths.

The creation of an individuated self, even the health of body and soul, is in the telling of our tales. Open to your stories. Say, sing, wail, dance, paint, write what you know to be your truth. "Mythology is the song, it is the song of the imagination inspired by the energies of the body," says Joseph Campbell. Let your stories meet and sing and dance with those of others, now and of the ancients, recognizing the eternal pulse that moves within, without, and among us as we breathe into the splits of soul and body.

167

And so it is that words and seeds become incarnate in the deep and dark feminine of instinct and Earth, where Snake sheds its skin and renewal emerges from loss. In the wisdom of her croning years, Lois Harvey reminds me that in my spiritual journey: "There is a rebirth of what has been lost. Only the form has changed."*

---

*Personal conversation, 1996.

new beginning
for my mother

We talk of a black woman who sells blackberry
pie at the farmer's market
when we drive downtown. At the play you are
ready to leave at intermission
back to your bed at the Hampton

dreams take you away
new worlds
open
silent bodies
float
in caves spoons
carved from
wood.

This is your destiny: harvest your soul!

Earlier in the day we sat together
fed our souls
poetry
story
my voice
yours

a new beginning
hearts open
read to me as
you have always
done.

—your son, David

INTO THE DARK
FOR GOLD

On a crisp fall weekend, J. Linn and I gathered in our mountain home with two other married couples—Pat and Bill, John and Lynn—to support and nurture our relationships as sacred in a context of love for creation, for our marriages, and for one another. My pulse quickened poignantly as we invoked the directions in the Indian way, as is our custom, sage smoke encircling our bodies as the beat of the drum called to the beat of our hearts. My heart, our hearts, the great heart containing us as an experience in the mind and heart of God.

I called to the Mother of Earth to join our circle and receive us, but words of invocation choked in my throat. Since J. Linn and I had taken our grownup children to see *Phantom of the Opera* some weeks earlier, I had frequently been on the verge of tears. I recognized my anguish in the phantom's wails, his tortured body moving with constraint while deepening him emotionally.

Sharing this experience, my friends encouraged me to express the emotion I had been suppressing. Even before I was conscious of having made any choice to share my pain, muscles that had been holding back feelings surrendered to the trust of our group. A deep and potent surge of energy moved in my body, and with my mind's eye I saw the image of a volcano, its power pushing up through rock, cracking the earth open with boiling lava.

From her underworld domain, Ereshkigal was asserting her presence right into the light of day. Like a train barreling at top speed through a long, dark tunnel, my energy thundered and expanded. I felt as if I had become the train, every throttle wide open and speeding along. I felt train power clear down to my toes. And Ereshkigal was the engineer.

We sped down the tracks, roaring and screaming with years of imprisoned suffering. Rage exploded from within my flesh. Venom overflowed my pores and oozed out everywhere, even from beneath my fingernails. Primal, wordless screams rebelled against my fate— subhuman sounds, intense wails unchained at last to express my repressed fury. My darkness burst into consciousness, and it did not feel like madness. Defeated? No. In grief, I felt empowered. Soon came words:

"No. NO. *NO!*" I exploded. "I reject this affliction. I hate it. I despise it. I loathe it! Take it away. Get it *off* me. Away! Away! I will not have it. GNAH AHHHHAAAA."

Sobbing, I went on: "I hate this illness. I'm sick and tired of trying to transform it into a gift. I work with it constantly. There's no gold." My cry went out to Mother Earth: "Why have you betrayed me?" I was surprised to feel this betrayal and to hear my own words. "Why? I've been a faithful daughter. Why, *why* have you turned away from me and left me unprotected? Reverently, I have cared for you. I've loved you with my whole heart. I love you still. I have tilled your soil with tenderness, mulched your dirt until it is brown and loamy. Lovingly, I tuck seeds into your open flesh. I've adorned you with beautiful flowers. I've been a devoted daughter, and you betray me. You abandon me. Why? Why?" Exhausted and crying quietly, I lay on the floor to rest.

A faint voice from Earth responded deep within me, "My child, my child. Oh, my dear child. I am so sorry you must go through this. As you suffer, I, too suffer. For you, my own tears drop.

"This is life's way. It is your turn. Let your tears flow and your rage be heard. Your dreams are crushed and your sorrow deep. I am with you. I see your tears and hear your painful groans. Together, we will comfort your despair. I will rock you gently for you dwell in the quietness of my own heart." Minutes of silence ensued.

"I can hear you," I responded eventually. "That helps. I don't understand. I try to transform the negativity into useful learnings."

Then I spoke to the Parkinson's: "What do you want from me? What do you require? Why have you come? Why do you torment me—searing my flesh with your madness?"

The illness replied: "I am opening you to the inward depths of your soul, to what matters, to make a space within you for a relationship with God. Even now, you and the Mother of Earth offer consolation and hope to one another. And there is more . . .."

"The light and the dark of who you are is no longer hidden. The opposites are revealed. You are not trying to live up to other people's expectations as before, and you are no longer withholding the fullness of who you are. We're getting to what's true for you as you meet yourself with acceptance instead of judgment."

"These are matters of body, heart, and soul that create the growing edge for your later years in life. When you accept all that is you, including even your own dying, there will be no more fear."

I challenged: "But why do I have to learn these things now? It's too early."

Silence. A while later, Parkinson's said, "You are past mid life, you are again in transition as you integrate being closer to death than childhood. You are about becoming more truly who you are, reuniting with the light and the dark parts of your psyche."

"There is a new life of wholeness that you can only now imagine. Be open, as a child is open. Allow the mystery in. This way of being is the way of growth. When you cover up your vulnerability, you shut out the sacred."

I wept. "That's true. That's true. I feel so ashamed when I need help walking or when my moving about is impaired. When medication is 'off,' I'm horrified at the old woman I may suddenly become.

"I try to stay in the moment, not daring to look ahead at the future. At the end of the day when I've taken my last medication, the drop from 'on' to 'off' is raw. I feel exposed, stripped of all dignity, as if I'm sinking into weakness that will shatter me utterly."

Parkinson's reassured me, "Like the Navajo rug woven with an imperfection in the corner where the Spirit moves in and out, you need me to open you up. Don't get hung up on past regrets and guilts. Nobody is keeping score. I am not a punishment. I am a wounding because

I want to be in your heart. When you suffer, you are vulnerable and I can be close to you.

"That's true for others, too. When you share the gift of your naturalness, your authenticity of self, you know the fulfillment of finding gold in this darkness. You also discover that you are coming to the wisdom of your croning years."

Through this exchange and other experiences, I am learning that we change destiny by bringing forth the fearful darkness we have repressed—the negative, shameful, embarrassing parts of ourselves. For me, I especially fear and hide my shame, my rage, and my despair.

Instead of rejecting these parts, I must bring them into awareness. Not doing so attracts negative energy to me in the visible world. The psyche's nature is to seek a balance of opposites in its journey to wholeness. So, unless I embrace my own undesired parts and create wholeness in my inner life, my psyche finds and attracts similarly undesired experiences and energies in the outer world. My growth and understanding are not by conscious choice, mind you. Fate has forced change upon me, and there's no going back. After fueling my earlier years, the draw of competition and public acclaim has now waned. I rarely feel driven. Ego is stepping aside to make way for the self to experience and express pain that was suffocating my soul.

As the intensity of my catharsis subsided, I heard my husband's cries. Our eyes met in both misery and compassion. With strong masculine support, Bill and John had moved behind and beside him as dear Pat and Lynn consoled me. J. Linn and I reached for one another, tears rolling down our cheeks, our hearts breaking open with grief as we lovingly embraced Parkinson's and each other. As our friends rocked us in a nest of comforting arms, we wept and then rested, singing: *Amazing grace, how sweet the sound that saved a soul like me.*

THE WORLD BENEATH
THE WORLD

"Mommy, Mommy . . . Where are you, Mommy? . . . Oh, Mommy, where are you?

In the dark of night I awaken, startled to hear the whimpering of a very young girl. Where is she, this child crying in the night? As consciousness rolls back the thick shades of sleep, I realize it is my own voice. These are the whimpers of my child self instinctively calling for the comfort of my mother in her eldering years of wisdom and for the Divine Mother, the Mother of God, the

Mami—a Sumerian name for she who is the origin and home of us all. To her, the feminine side of God, I call out in my deepest vulnerability.

For those of us contending with fear and emotional or physical pain, it is neither unusual nor abnormal to feel exposed, like a tree stripped of its protective bark, or a turtle without its shell. Naturally, we may regress to the vulnerability of the childhood self, the self we knew before we developed our ego precautions and protections. For me, even nerve endings become overly sensitive to sound.

Hearing my inner child cry out that night took me to an acutely vulnerable feeling. In my imagination, I reached out and gathered her into the safety of my arms, holding her to my heart as the maternal part of my psyche sought to comfort the child part. Somehow, that helped.

Similar difficult times sometimes come in the night. When my life's loss and deprivation crowd out stamina and spontaneity, intimations of disablement, suffering, and even death stalk my sleepless hours. Who am I now? Who am I becoming? Chronic illness and incriminating signs of aging thrust me into transition and change without any map of this threatening terrain or signposts along the way to reassure me that others have also survived the travel. I remind myself that the old way of being must give way, even die, to make room for a new flowering of wisdom and creativity in my croning years, for this is the life–death–rebirth cycle of the feminine.

Allowing new possibilities to emerge and take shape transforms that which I have lost.

Cutting new paths through the dense and dark forest of illness and aging makes pioneers of us all. Both experiences are individualized, with new role models and no tried-and-true trails. We must create our own guideposts, improvising as we go, step by painful step. Moving into the shadows, we call instinctively to our original mother. We reach for her, and in response she draws us into her depths.

As night weaves its tenuous way to dawn spontaneous chants and the verses of hymns learned in childhood as a minister's daughter slip into my consciousness. They appear in my memory as guides through lonely times, preserved precisely as I committed them to memory originally. With unwavering childlike trust and faith in their power, I want to sing from my bed into the night. Hymn after hymn and verse upon verse, they join together as beads on a thread, radiating peace like the prayers of a rosary. I am blessed by the comfort they bring and thankful for the importance they have always held for my family.

When music fills my body and soul with the vibration of life, I make less room for fearing my illness. Relatives and friends applaud the strength of my confident self, who guides my days as I cope with Parkinson's and even lets me forget temporarily that the defenseless-child aspect huddles in my psyche's shadows, symbolizing helplessness as well as hope.

Each year also brings new increments of the emerging crone, the wise old woman, bearer of life's healing opportunities and death's mysterious presence. For her as well as for the mother and the maiden, life's possibilities and limitations coexist in the same moment of suffering. They "open us to our own center," write Massimilla and Bud Harris in their empowering book *Like Gold Through Fire* (p. 83):

> and allow for a third position filled with new
> life which today we cannot even imagine. And
> this is the mystery. That by participating in the
> great unknowns we are able to become at home

in a dreadful world and discover the deeper
pulse of life.

Whatever our call to fate—be it impairment, relocation, aging, estrangement, addiction, depression, death,
or something else—it precipitates crisis as the hardy ego
collapses. Fate is an alien intruder and an agent of change
who plunges us into turmoil and chaos—into a world
beneath the world, seething with energy that both
destroys and regenerates. We often feel terrified and
out of control, desperate to maintain order and a sembl-
ance of the *status quo* in life as we have known it.

For those of us whose struggle includes making the
archetypal journey to the soul, the crisis may invite us

down into the dark and chaotic unconscious of our primal nature. That descent entails leaving the familiar to venture into the region of shadows, into which we have repressed various experiences and their accompanying feelings, and to which we have exiled parts of our personalities that we deem shameful and unacceptable. Severed from the *status quo ante,* we proceed down and down, aware that destiny has us in its grip while, as someone once said, life wobbles and then falls to dust as we descend into the dark where all possibilities of life and death are contained.

We are drawn to the hidden and unseen, to a crossroads where the four directions converge and where opposites must contend for dominance. Those cutoff, denied aspects of ourselves have gathered energy in the unconscious like roots and tendrils that proliferate and extend until strong enough to challenge the surface. Hecate, the old and wise woman of Greek mythology, guides us as we descend into our fears while "tears fall to form a stream of holy water that will flow beside us until our sorrowing is complete."* These enlightened words of Clarissa Estes call us to mourn as life moves through us. Change brings loss, and with loss come our tears of grief as we recognize our wounds and grieve for our own hearts. According to a Sufi verse, "When the heart weeps for what it has lost, the soul rejoices for what it has found."

---

*Women Who Run with the Wolves, p. 423.

This paradox connects to the idea that the netherworld's dreadful chaos contains hidden patterns of creation that connect us to some greater spirit as we make meaning of our lives and expand into possibilities theretofore unimagined. For instance, images from the unconscious carry healing powers if we open to receive their creative infusion. My own dreams bring me various images of descent, including mine shafts or caves deep in the earth, the unfathomable depths of the ocean, or the belly of a goose.

The process of dreaming and then working to understand my dreams is deep nourishment that transforms my life and brings hope. Like a loving mother, my dreams mirror the psyche's deep feelings with compassion and offer new possibilities for continuing my ordeal. Using the image of wilderness, Marion Woodman and Elinor Dickson describe part of this process of understanding as a "place of reckoning." In their words,*

>the wilderness conjures up images of danger, isolation, and aloneness. Physically, it is the place where we meet ourselves, undistracted by people or events. We are alone. All our fears rise up to meet us. We are tested to the utmost. If we can endure the terror, the wilderness also becomes a place where we can begin to experience our own strength, our own resources, and

---

Dancing in the Flames, pp. 119-120.

our own truth. The gospels record that following his baptism, Christ, too, was drawn into the wilderness, where he confronted the temptations of his shadow demon and overcame them.

We recognize the experience of the wilderness in our own lives: a severe illness, the death of a loved one, the breakdown of a marriage, the loss of a job, the shaking of our faith, the shock of realizing our own limitations. These places are wilderness because they isolate us so that we cannot be reached by the outside world. These experiences we ultimately have to go through alone. Others may be present on the periphery, but it is as if a veil descends between us and them, leaving us alone, to struggle by and with ourselves.

The image of wilderness emerged in my dreams and connected powerfully to my situation with Parkinson's.

> I dream that the living room of my house opens into a wilderness with wild and treacherous terrain. There is no doorway, wall, or boundary to delineate the living area of the house from the dangers of the outside. Suddenly, a panther springs from a ledge to attack a deer. Their struggle is brief as the panther hungrily rips the warm flesh from the bones of the deer. I feel endangered, attacked, and sad.

My living room represents the space in which I live, where normalcy and dangers exist side by side. At times,

I feel as if Parkinson's pounces on me like this dream's panther attacking and dismembering her prey. The deer embodies my losses, activities, and strengths—which at times my condition seems to be striping from me, one by one.

Yet, this wilderness is not toxic. Both panther and deer are strong, vital, beautiful creatures that we can view as participating in the eternal pattern of life–death–rebirth. The deer's life may provide sustenance for the panther to nourish her young, for panthers are known to kill only when hungry.

In this dream, I witness the mysterious pattern of affinities that connects me to all of life, each of us destined to play a part in the cosmic story. Primal peoples knew this well. They offered rituals of appreciation to the spirit of any animal slain to feed the tribe. When I see the dream in this way, I too, participate in the archetypal story of life and in that experience is meaning, even awe. When my personal story connects to universal truth, my shock at recognizing that truth draws me into the presence of the sacred, where I feel valued by healing archetypal dimensions.

The following dream is one of transformation in which Eros, ancient Greek god of love, emerges from the integration of domination and submission.

Dreamlight
1996

> Later the same night, I dream of being at the entrance of a large cave, peering into its darkness. In the shadows, I see humanlike

figures gliding by quietly. They seem to have no
delineated features and move gracefully. I strain
to see more as I move into the cave and am
drawn toward a dim light ahead and to the left.

This cave is like a sanctuary, a cathedral. Reverence and hushed words now follow the bold dream of the panther and deer. I see a diffuse light on the left, the side that Eastern spiritual thought designates as the body's unconscious and feminine side. The dream's figures are not limited to embodied life. They move with grace, gliding effortlessly, unlike the awkward movement I often experience. When medication imbalance causes dyskenesia, my limbs may move erratically. These fluid dream figures seem to be from beyond this world, perhaps spirit figures letting me know I am not alone.

Dreamlight
1996

I have arrived in a new community. As I approach the center of the town, the plaza, I see a magnificent totem or scepter. It is a long-handled spoon carved into the trunk of a living tree and oiled to a rich and moist finish so as to accentuate the beauty of the grain visible in the wood. This beauty and the meaning of the totem so touch my heart that I weep copiously. I call the people of the town together and discover that the artist is a middle-aged woman with curly hair. She is unaware of the importance of her contribution. I announce to the townspeople that this totem heralds a new ruling principle for their lives. Because this is a spoon, a symbol of nourishment, carved into a living tree, a symbol of the feminine—instead of a sword, symbol of masculine authority—there will never be domination in this town, only the love of equality. My tears continue to flow as the crowd cheers and people embrace one another.

In the next scene, I see a sleeping child, a girl about six or seven years old. I know that it is my responsibility to lead her home to her people. To do this, we must make our way through a dark forest. I awaken her gently and we start off, hand in hand. To me, she is light and wonder. As we enter the forest, she transforms into the woman who carved the totem. We try to find the key or pitch that is comfortable for both of us to sing the well-loved

spiritual "There is a Balm in Gilead." I know
that this prayerful sharing of our voices will
strengthen us on our journey to her tribe.

As Michelangelo could see life in stone, so the wise
woman of my dream brings forth the beauty of the inner
nature beneath the wood's grain. As the tree of life's
branches reach toward heaven and its roots press deep
into the richness of underworld potentialities, this symbol of individuation joins with spirit. It is Eros, rather
than patriarchy, who now rules. My soul self, the deeper
self within, unites the mature creatress and the inno-
cent child, and the light and dark of all that I am—one
polarity containing the other—as we find our way
through the cycles of Earth to the center. It is right that

this soul child finds her roots, her people, here in this land of trees, this forest.

What does it mean for my life that Eros rules the land? Welcoming the god of love first brings forth all in me that is not loving, all that is not nice. It brings me face to face with my shadow, my darkness, my worst fears. Repression's curtain opens to reveal the humiliations of illness, the cold and stark silence of loneliness, and the nauseating pain of violence; my jealousy, envy, and rage; the shameful out-of-control helplessness of my own human need; and the deep sorrowing of betrayal. The love of Eros offers safety for confessing the torments of my soul.

Rather than denying or cursing my symptoms, I must kiss the frog. To transform the ignored and loathed into the fullness of being alive means making room in my heart for all that I am, including my symptoms and torments, even when the infinite comes to me in the form of Parkinson's in the prime of my life.

And this is the sacrifice. I must abandon all hope of mobilizing heroic efforts to rise willfully above the realities of my situation. For my soul and body's sake, I must soften my heart to receive my own flesh. What has been hard and hardened, judged and judgmental must now soften for me to welcome it fully. To do so is to accept mercifully that my power is limited and my need deep.

Rigid attachments to performance, excellence, and ego successes give way to making my descent into the deep and dark world beneath the world. Only when I face myself with radical honesty am I free to grow and change—to heal into the joys and celebrations in the completeness of my own nature. What I retrieve can then emerge from the shadow.

The spoon in my dream points to nourishment given and received spoonful by spoonful, sip by sip, step by step. Rather than the gulping down of food, the spoon is suggestive of small portions that I can taste, chew, digest, and integrate. Both overfeeding and underfeeding result in malnourishment; not so with the spoon. The spoon's sculptress shows that something new is available now and that townspeople are ready to take in this nourishment. That is, they are ready to assimilate it and become conscious so that growth and change may bring new life day by day, spoonful by spoonful, in the miracle of creation. I have learned that a full life is lived moment by moment. Being present in the moment—that is, attentive and intentional—I discover I am already prepared for what lies ahead.

I think it is a Yiddish story that speaks of souls who gathered in the dining hall of heaven. There they found tables of sumptuous food and long-handled spoons. Try as they might, it was simply impossible to get those spoons to their mouths. Fortunately, a creative soul came up with the idea that the spoons would work quite well if they fed one another. And so they did.

> There is a balm in Gilead to make the wounded whole.
>
> There is a balm in Gilead to heal the lonely soul.
>
> Sometimes I feel discouraged and think my work's in vain.
>
> But then the Holy Spirit revives my soul again.*

---

*"There Is a Balm in Gilead," *The Presbyterian Hymnal*, p. 396.

OF ONE HEART

Having heard that traditional peoples sometimes dig holes in the earth to fill with the tears and wails of their sorrows, I knelt and dug my hole in the garden one day, soggy soil making mud spots on the knees of my jeans. Then I stretched full length on the earth, placing my cheek upon the lap of God, and waited . . . dry-eyed and numb. Nothing. Only the heaviness in my heart, my creative pulse stilled.

> Oh, Mary! Don't cha weep? Don't cha mourn?
> Oh, Mary, Mother of God, won't cha weep?
> Won't cha mourn?

Turning over and over in my mind, Gayle Jackson's voice moans with the refrains of spirituals. Melody lines sing themselves while my body presses into the Earth's moist body. Mendelssohn slips almost unnoticed into my awareness.

> Oh, rest in the Lord.
> Wait patiently for Him.
> And He shall give you your heart's desire.
> And he shall give you your heart's desire.
> Oh, Mary, yes, you weep. Yes, you mourn.

My mother in her later years seizes life with the energy and brilliance of a very young woman. With a loving spirit, she welcomes family and friends into her heart and hearth. And in her presence, we are nourished. I have noticed a deepened sweetness in the love my mother and father share, fragrant with the bloom of youth and ripe with the mellowing of growing old. Dysfunction and early-life wounds, the grist for growth in all relations, dissolve into love. The cherishing of one another is what matters now.

Day after day, my mother waits patiently upon my father. Only remnants are left of the scholar he once was, reminding us of another life that once thrived. Dwelling in a body declining with years and Alzheimer's gives him the prerogative of letting anyone be who he needs her to be—the nurse, a daughter; the daughter, a sister, aunt, or friend—as he tries to gather together the pieces and people of his life as heirlooms. Lucidity and confusion vie for the spaces of his mind that concentration and memory once inhabited. "Pray for those," requests my mother, "for whom memory no longer serves well."

One morning he asks, "Is this death? Didn't we die in Burgaw?"

"Oh, no, my love, this is a hospital. We're quite alive. We went to high school in Burgaw." Then she asks gently, "Are you thinking about death today?"

My father nods, "Who will be waiting for me?"

With the wisdom so like my mother, she intuitively connects him to his own depths. "Now, who would you like to be waiting for you?"

"Mama." he replies.

"And what would you like to tell your mama?"

His face glowing with love, my father looks directly at my mother, certain in that moment that she is his wife of nearly sixty years, and says, "I want to tell Mama that living my life with you was heaven on earth."

Oh, Mary, don't cha weep. Don't cha mourn. Oh, Mary! He plunged right into the love. The song of triumph has begun. He's following his life right into his heart.

Telling me about this later, my mother's voice shimmered with the joy of a maiden in love. My body stirs as I hear the faint, deep moan of my soul. My father is dying. My father is dying. A wail of loss and a song of joy merge as tears and laughter water my soul. His dying, my dying, the dying of us all—we are of one heartbeat. I weep with gratitude for the life of my father and this moment of fullness.

After that, peace seemed to radiate through the family, even for those of us hundreds of miles away. Matters of the heart have no time or distance. That day, death became—for me, and perhaps for others—part of living, part of the one process of dying and being reborn moment by moment by moment. I felt no fear, only a seamless garment in which life and death were one in a space called love.

THE LABYRINTH
BENEATH OUR FEET

We had come to Ghost Ranch, all forty of us, diverse in age and spiritual practice. There, at this Presbyterian conference center nestled in the high desert of New Mexico, terra cotta canyon walls and forms of rock and shale etched like hieroglyphics create cathedrals in the natural world, luminous and forever. The evening sun seemed to empty itself of glimmering ribbons which danced against the gathering dark as we turned to one another, curious about how and why each had felt drawn to this remote place.

We had signed up for a week-long workshop led by Lauren Artress, an Episcopal priest, to walk the Ghost Ranch labyrinth. Since antiquity, spiritual pilgrims have used this archetypal meditative device to lead themselves to the sacred center of their souls. The geometry of Ghost Ranch's healing maze replicates a labyrinth laid in tiles 800 years ago on the floor of the cathedral in Chartres, France to honor Mary, Mother of God.

Truly, the labyrinth is a metaphor for life and the search for spirit. Thirsting for God involves leaving the familiar to walk an unknown path. It means turning to the shadows to see ourselves more completely, to face our lives more honestly, and to bring into conscious light that which we have kept hidden, especially from ourselves.

I was glad to be sharing the experience with J. Linn, despite his reservations about being one of only four men among thirty-six women. He and I spoke of feeling anxious as we anticipated walking this ancient pattern of seekers. I also worried about whether I could physically walk the labyrinth's lengthy spiral path, which wound imposingly over many feet of canvas.

Clearly, I wanted to tell the group about having Parkinson's. Only then could I bring my full energy to walking the labyrinth without being preoccupied about moving awkwardly. Again and again, I find that when I acknowledge my truth openly, more of me becomes available for coping with my challenges. It also relieves me of any need to hide my symptoms.

As it turned out, the first walk was scheduled at night, when I am not sure-footed enough to walk distances unaided. So I prepared instead to walk early the next morning. Meanwhile, watching the group's night walk, I saw a blind woman resting her hands on the shoulders of her dear friend as they slowly made their way with care-filled steps to the center of the labyrinth. I felt deeply moved.

The following morning, drawing silence around me and focusing on the gentle rhythm of my breathing, I stepped expectantly upon the path. From the outside edge to the compelling core, I walked the serpentine way, step after step, sometimes approaching the center, sometimes wandering away.

As I walked, concerns regarding the outer world slipped away, leaving space for something new to manifest. After several hours on the path, however, something puzzled me. I seemed fully alert and present as I walked, yet I felt nothing. I received nothing. No new longed-for insight, no strong emotion, no words of wisdom from my unconscious appeared. No nugget of gold emerged to contemplate. I felt as dry as the *arroyos* in the desert that surrounded us. Whether I was pre-occupied about being physically able to walk the labyrinth or whether I feared what might be revealed to me, I do not know.

How was I blocking my responsiveness? I heard the critical voice of judgment within, cawing like a crow. "See, you can't do this right. You might as well hang it up, forget it. You're a fool to hope for new awareness. You've had all the healing you're going to get."

Fortunately, my wise intuition spoke up: "OK, Les, so you don't feel anything, no problem. How do you feel about feeling nothing?"

Like an earthquake, I felt the ground beneath me sway as emotions quickly rose. "Angry! That's what I feel. I feel *ANGRY!* Maybe there really is no more help for me? Do I expect too much? My God, don't forsake me again!" I wanted to pound my fists into the labyrinth's pathway. Lurking within my anger, these lies—that my healing was over, that I would receive no more help—tormented me. Behind the terror of my situation that surged, I also felt life's power enlivening my body and soul through my anger.

Without restraint, I wept and I wailed until a familiar subtle shift occurred. This somehow happens whenever I permit myself to dip into my deepest, most gut-wrenching emotions. As if responding to a preset course, my anger and fear transform into deep sadness. In that sadness, as I allow myself to breathe and receive comfort, I discover great relief. That day at Ghost Ranch, as he has over the years, J. Linn bore unflinching witness to the sounds of my suffering by remaining calmly and quietly present. He reminded me to feel the tension of opposing feelings that moved through me.

Beyond the silence I encountered in the labyrinth, I was finding life's force in my rage and empowerment in my grief. My fear of disability was leading me to a deep sadness that softened and opened my heart to receive an infusion of love for myself and all life. Consciously, I struggled to hold onto my despair and in the same moment its opposite, the yearning to heal, as I sensed intimations of something else stirring. A new level of knowing, a fresh awareness, was being born through my sorrow.

Pressing into my consciousness was a reconnection to all of life, with its joy and its terrible pain. Momentarily, it was as if I became all things organic: human, animal, and plant. The web of life called to me through vibrating cells that respond to one another over time, species, and space.

My personal experience was swirling into a bigger story. Its full revelation became clearer the following day, when J. Linn and I drove out across the desert in search of a Benedictine community of monks well noted for their chanting. Arriving at their rustic sanctuary in time for choir practice, we welcomed the deep comfort of their singing. A nearby statue of Mary drew me to light some candles. I knelt at her feet, then wept my prayers for healing. I longed for a new awareness, a fresh perspective, connection with the holy feminine.

With every step on the labyrinth's path, I had looked and listened within, searching for the expressions of my own nature, my truth as a woman with disability. I had found feelings that fueled my subjective world and that were pushing me to express them openly, without shame and embarrassment, but I had not experienced the solace I found at the feet of Mary.

Our visit to the Benedictine community was on the eve of the celebration of Mary's assumption, a day that sanctifies and raises her to inclusion in the godhead as Queen of Heaven, the divine image of woman, a woman God, mother of earth and sky. Her assumption honors all women who long to reclaim their divinity. For men with that longing, it honors the feminine in them—the capacity to share matters of the heart and body: feelings, relatedness, the fecundity and moistness of the natural world, the details and ordinariness of life made holy.

In our deepest feeling experience, God incarnates in us. Changing, pulsating, struggling, emerging, evolving— through our struggles, the tears of our labors, and the longings of our hearts, God gives authentic voice to what we know is real. Through our woundedness, God is being born in us.

As we shed tears for the sufferings of all who have ever felt devalued, we hear the call to authenticity.

Reaching into our deepest injury, we meet the feminine face of God, who lifts us up to the holy. In consciousness, we bring that divine presence into the psyche, where it remains, ever present yet invisible. In consciousness, we lean into the eternal nearness of God the Mother.

For centuries, traditional peoples have turned to the east each morning to witness the rising sun, believing their participation is needed to call it up. If they do not turn toward the east—that is, to God the Mother/Father—no sons or daughters will rise to fulfill their deepest yearnings for the holy. Such people respect their own divinity.

After visiting the monastery, walking the labyrinth became a celebration for me. I had learned that I must yet again experience my shadow before I am ready to receive the light of grace. It is, after all, the way of the feminine to include the completeness of who we are— the parts and pieces, rejected and broken; fragments that reveal our wounds and shortcomings; and aspects that we have yet to develop. Even aspects that express anger and rage.

At Ghost Ranch, I felt part of the sky's expansive stretch to embrace the receptive Earth, and a part of Earth's surrender of her gaze heavenward. The vast New Mexico sky never seems to cease wooing Earth. The power and holiness of the place had energized, opened, and deepened me. And the people who gathered there had blessed my life. I wanted to run, to skip, and to dance with joy through the labyrinth. And I did!

Returning home to North Carolina, I remembered weeks later that in Chartres, above the labyrinth's tiled floor, a magnificent rose window depicts Mary ascending into heaven. The labyrinth beneath my feet, the spirit of woman rising.

FEATHERING
THE SOUL

For nine years now, he has come. With the advent of spring, I imagine the wood thrush preparing for flight from his winter home in the rain forest across the Gulf of Mexico to his summer home in my back yard. After nearly a decade, the reliable rhythm of his journey and appearance are well integrated in my annual anticipation. We are linked, he and I, in the invisible pulse of life: he delights my spirit with *jouissance* for three brief months, and I hear him into song. His visit completes with summer's first shift into fall.

Like a thirsty child, I wait eagerly each summer dawn for my feathered friend to come to the tree outside my bedroom window to sing up the sunrise, his rhapsodic sound bringing me to a new day where I have never been. How he returns to that tree year after year is one of life's miracles. The wonder I feel reminds me of the little girl I used to be: delighted with soft grass and pictures in clouds, my boundaries surrendering to the natural world that held me then as now.

Sickness catapults me into the stark recognition of life's fragility: that flesh is the lesson we have come to learn. Intrusively, the future calls for contemplation. And as I reluctantly peek from present toward what is yet to come, I see the inevitability of dying. Perhaps one of chronic illness's strange gifts is that it calls me to inward attentiveness, where who I am and who I was born to be are utterly important. Where everything is changed from profane to holy. For one breathless moment, archetypal love brings me to the point of stillness, punctuated by tears, where boundaries melt into the center of the one soul to which we all belong. For me, that is where transformative healing occurs.

With heart and soul, I climb atop the mighty wings of my wood thrush, soaring like the spirit of holiness between heaven and earth.

> The lone wild bird in lofty flight
> Is still with Thee, nor leaves Thy sight.

229

And I am thine! I rest in Thee.
Great Spirit, come, and rest in me.*

The dark of earth and the light of spirit join divine and profane in a space of mystery where they rub against one another in love. And in the rubbing, as the feathers of the soul begin to sprout, a shiver of wholeness fills the moment.

Some say the soul is feathered so that when we feel a presence as if from beyond this life, goosebumps ripple on the skin. The glory of the soul has drawn near.

---

*"The Lone Wild Bird," *The Presbyterian Hymnal,* p. 320.

HER OWN WAY

Waiting in K-Mart's parking lot recently for J. Linn, I spied a woman pulling into the handicapped spot nearby. I became totally absorbed in watching her struggle to get out of her van and heave her body into walking motion. A little younger than I, she wore a brace on her shriveled left leg and a prosthetic right leg in a highly wedged shoe. "How does she bear the stares and whispers?" I wondered. "How does she bear the difficult strain of what it takes for her to move?"

Then, in my imagination, I slipped into her body, trying to feel what it must be like for her to live there. It was a strange experiment. And as I struggled with what I perceived her struggle must be like—in part, anyway— the beauty of her courage flooded my senses. Judgment and pity dissolved, replaced instantly by admiration and inspiration. Upright and walking by then, she was doing what most of us do every day—in her own way.

ADAPTATION

The muse of my music is my nighttime consort when sleep irregularities come with taking my meds. Hours of silence often roll by as I serenade the night into dawn, singing every song I can recall and then making up my own. It's important to get more into the singing and less into the clock beside the bed, which today shows 5 A.M. when I awake after slumbering most of the night.

I even remember my dreams this morning, and they aren't horror scenes of being pursued, violated, hunted down, or any of the other umpteen metaphors that represent feeling victimized by my illness.

**Dreamlight
1998**

> I find a smaller house with a beautiful reddish-brown carpet that is old and evGen patched in places but clearly usable and appealing. Clean, large windows open onto a lush, wooded scene. I am delighted with my discovery.

Like the smaller house, my life is limited, made smaller by Parkinson's, yet I can feel open and expansive, continuing to grow.

My feet have not yet begun to cramp this morning. If I can just close my eyes and lie ever so still, maybe I can ward off the daily attack of dystonia, or muscle cramps. Muscles depleted of dopamine sometimes twist and writhe like snakes in a lair. The first time it happened, I awoke into pain and terror. Now this symptom is part of moving into the day. I tell myself it's only discomfort. Stay relaxed. Breathe deeply. Let the sensation float on through. Try not to brace against it.

Acceptance instead of judgment helps in many situations. Rather than labeling dystonia as painful and dreaded, I simply try to notice this or that sensation as it happens. With practice, this often works.

By lying on my stomach across the foot of our bed with my feet hanging off in mid-air, I discover I can delay dystonia's onset. I think it has something to do with the pull of gravity and the weight of my feet. (Several years after I discovered this, the Johns Hopkins Medical Letter for October 1998 described this position as a viable treatment for the discomfort of dystonia. That validated trusting myself to create home remedies when possible.)

With a mild groan of sleepy protest, J. rolls into a modified fetal position diagonally across the bed. Our hands reach for and find each other again. As the pink sky embraces the east, I take solace in the regularity of nature's awakenings and listen for our wood thrush's song. At daybreak yesterday, for the first time this spring, I heard him singing his message of wonder. It was my birthday.

IT TAKES A TEAM

As small children, David and Tanya built elaborate structures with smooth, geometrically shaped wooden blocks, often extending beyond the boundaries of the room into the hall. Bickering abated as this joint project fully engaged both my children, despite their being four years apart in age. Squeals of completion and sighs of fulfillment heralded an invitation to view their amazing achievement.

The process seemed more important than the outcome in that once they finished a structure, I soon heard a thundering of wood as the walls came tumbling down. In the ensuing stillness, they undertook another architectural feat.

A new creation can happen only after the destruction of what has been. This is the rhythm of building up and taking down. Here's the rub: no new life can emerge without a death—a letting go, a release from what has been. Nowhere is this more apparent than in our gardens, where rotting leaves and withered blossoms nourish new plants that press through soil and rock to find their place in the sun. Life, death, and life's renewal—this cycle characterizes all that lives. It is the way of the feminine, which is the process of all change, whether we are ill or well.

Throughout my adaptation to an ongoing health challenge, some very practical, down-to-earth learnings about self-care have made my life easier. With thanks to Virginia Satir for these thoughts on integrating change, I offer them here with the hope that they may be useful to you or somebody you know with a chronic health condition.

Chaos is a good sign.

Chaos indicates being in transition, a process of change that has predictable stages. The shock of diagnosis

239

disturbs the status quo, the familiarity of routines, so that you and your loved ones may feel as if your lives have been turned upside down.

This chaos is inevitable—and necessary. To create something new, you are returning temporarily to the primal chaotic matrix of creative energy. The former order comes tumbling down, as it must, to make a space for new possibilities. The inevitable chaos is a sign that you are moving through this time of reorientation to a new, more current way of living.

Take baby steps.

During the chatoic phase, make immediate, short-term decisions only. Avoid big, long-range plans while you are in the chaotic phase of your healing. When you are in emotional upheaval and confusion, it is important to get centered, because crisis unbalances your life. It is crucial to establish a new center of gravity. This comes by taking small steps to find a new balance.

Remember to breathe.

Taking time to breathe deeply brings peace. Gradually, one moment to the next, you can learn to add new behaviors or adaptations that are more comfortable and fitting for your life now. In time, these new behaviors become as familiar as your previous ones.

Show yourself daily kindness.

Look each day for small ways to be kind to yourself, such as getting a massage or calling a faraway friend. Be gentle with yourself. You are not to blame because you have an illness. This is not a reprimand for wrongdoing. The purpose of your illness is not to punish you but to make love more manifest. Don't shut yourself out of your own heart.

Reach out and touch.

Touch heals. Get an infusion of endorphins daily. Virginia Satir would often say that we need at least twelve hugs a day to maintain health.

Eliminate all stress.

Eliminating stress means paying exquisite attention to your body–mind–spirit. They are one. Learn to recognize when you are reaching your limit, even with activities you enjoy. Ask yourself, "Is what I am doing now returning energy to me?" If it does not give back energy, consider doing something different. Stop while you are enjoying what is happening, not when you are depleted.

Focus on what you CAN do.

One way to live with less stress is to focus on what you *can* do rather than what you cannot do. It may well be that your best choice is to let the sun's rays caress you as you yield to one moment of your life at a time. Remember that creating a balanced self and world takes both extraverted "do-ers" as well as quiet, introverted "be-ers."

All your feelings matter.

All your feelings are normal, and they do matter. It is important to have a way of expressing them safely. Writing, drawing, or painting your feelings can be useful.

244

I know of nothing more healing than having another person who is receptive to your feelings and can listen with acceptance and without evaluation or judgment. A counselor, a member of the clergy, or trusted friend may be helpful. In most communities, support groups exist for patients with specific chronic conditions. Expressing and understanding feelings helps avert depression.

Get a specialist.

Even if your family doctor or general practitioner is monitoring your condition and medication, also seeing a specialist is worthwhile. In addition to their awareness

245

of cutting-edge research and developments in treating your condition, they bring special training and skills to managing the vagaries of your particular set of symptoms and daily rhythms. You, your medications, and your symptoms are like a dance team: subtle movements of sensitivity to one another create greater comfort, ease, and enjoyment for you. A specialist can lend expert direction to your own choreography.

A case in point is my neurologist and Parkinson's specialist, Dr. Kathleen Shannon. She is an artist when it comes to maximizing results from minimal changes in my medication. She also brings valuable skill to combining medications. Although I see her only two to four times a year, getting to Chicago has been well worth the effort.

Taking medication promptly is important, especially in chronic illness. My daughter, Tanya, and my son-in-law, Craig, found a wonderful gadget for me. It is a pocket-sized beeper and pill dispenser set for my schedule. It frees me from worry about remembering my medication hourly. For those of us who must take meds regularly with no extra time to spare, it is a treasure.

Take medication on time.

Try alternative treatments. In addition to allopathic (conventional Western) medicine, try alternative treatments. Be sure your practitioner has a written list of all medications, supplements and vitamins you are taking. It was Dr. Shannon who urged me to learn Tai Chi, a Chinese movement meditation effective for increasing balance. Every week, I also schedule three sessions of various alternative treatments that I find beneficial, including massage, cranial sacral treatment, Traeger bodywork, Feldenkreis movement work, Rubenfeld Synergy, chiropractic, hypnosis, and Chinese medicine.

As the oldest medical system in the world (2,500 years), Chinese medicine establishes balance and harmony within the body through the use of herbal medicine and acupuncture. Acupuncture regulates the body's flow of blood and *qi* (life force, pronounced *"chee"*). The doctor inserts sterile needles at certain acupoints to improve the flow and balance of energy.

I have been blessed to receive treatment from two highly skilled doctors of Oriental medicine: Phil Ricker, OMD, a well prepared, intently focused and deeply caring practitioner in Asheville, North Carolina; and Dianne Conelly, PH.D., OMD, dean of the Traditional Acupuncture Institute in Columbia, Maryland. She creatively and compassionately combines a psycho-spiritual process with her gifts and expertise in the practice of acupuncture as she brings her patients "home" to their own hearts.

My view is that Chinese medicine offers a highly effective approach to treating my illness and nourishing my health when used in partnership with Western medicine. I brew and drink a tea of Chinese herbs before each meal and receive acupuncture every other week. As a result, I feel stronger, have a greater sense of well being, suffer fewer "on" or "off" fluctuations, sleep more soundly, and have been able to reduce other medication.

Keep moving.

If you have a movement challenge, moving is as important as your medication. Playing music with a strong beat may help you move more easily. Music that pleases you heals.

One of my greatest pleasures is turning on one of Aretha Franklin's CDs of gospel music on high volume. I sing and dance till no breath is left in me. Rebecca Wells in *Little Altars Everywhere* (p. xii) says it with zest:

> something secret, something sweet, something strong, is shooting up from the earth straight into my body making my limbs quiver, making me crazy dance all over the place . . ..

251

**Find the
presence
of the
divine.**

In my experience, connecting with the divine is most important. Find a way to see your condition as a spiritual path. Linking your situation to a larger perspective helps you find meaning for your life. Your illness can then become a quest for deepened growth. Meditation, prayer, visualizations and hypnosis work. Each practice seeks to develop focus and heightened awareness not ordinarily accessible in daily activities. It is the realm of deep and alert relaxation that bypasses ego, limitations, and activates regions of the mind for healing self and others.

Ideally, your life partner can share your journey on a spiritual level. If not, you may find friends who can.

You may find therapeutic growth groups, religious groups organized to deal with issues of grief and loss, or support groups for people in transition.

Ill or well, we all need a support team. This certainly holds true when we face special challenges. When I pull away from loved ones to protect them from my physical and emotional discomfort, I've learned, they may feel shut out and rejected. By gently insisting on being with me in rough times, my close friends and family have

Let those who love you care for you.

253

reminded me of the healing comfort and deep connection that comes when I share my greatest vulnerabilities.

The following visualizing exercise was inspired by Virginia Satir's Parts Party, a therapeutic intervention using psychodrama to acknowledge and integrate parts of the personality. (Unless your memory is quite good, you may want to tape-record it initially so you can go through the steps without needing to stop and refer back to each one.) Take your time. Proceed slowly and pause often.

Find a way to be as comfortable as possible where you sit or lie. This is a time to relax, so take a deep, nourishing breath through your nose and, as you exhale through your mouth, release any tightness or tension. Again, a deep nose breath followed by a full exhalation. Take as much time as you like. [Pause.]

On the next exhalation, allow your eyes to close gently. Imagine being in a beautiful natural setting. It may be a place you know or have visited, or it may be a place you create in your imagination right now. [Pause.]

When you have that scene in mind imagine that your friends, family members, and other loved ones are gathering to visit with you. Include in this gathering all who are important to you—your doctors, support people, caretakers, and especially your pets. Take as much or as little time as you need to greet each one as she or he arrives.

Now allow these people who care for you to gather into a circle of love, with you in the middle. One by one, each then comes to stand next to you and, gently resting a hand on your body in a loving and comfortable way, speaks a few words of care to you. In your imagination, allow each to give you a message, such as "I bring you the gift of courage." One might offer words of appreciation or love. Another might say simply, "I'm glad we're friends."

Imagine these people's gentle, non-invasive touch to convey meaning as you feel each person's hand resting on your body in a caring way and hear love in the sound of each voice. In this way, let the light of their souls shine on you. Let yourself soften to receive their love for you. Let it flow over you like a gentle mountain waterfall. The imprint of their voices and touch will remain in your body and heart always, even as their hands move away.

When you are ready, let the scene fade from imagination as you take a deep breath and open your eyes.

When I do this exercise, I usually feel strengthened and supported. From within a deep space of emotional openness, endless love and trust lifts me up to the level of the eternal, the realm of archetypal power, where healing of miraculous proportions sometimes occurs.

WHOLE AND HOLY

In these wild and venerable mountains of North Carolina, I have taken root. I have come to love Earth deeply,
experiencing her as both radiant and vicious, feeling her
great comforting lap holding me with gravity, knowing
in my bones that she is the source of my origins and the
home of my endings. Alpha and Omega. She is Earth
Mother, known as Gaia, who within her body contains
all that lives and all that dies. It is she who generously
provides the bounty to sustain our bodies, the beauty

that nourishes the soul, and the power to wail forth the blizzards of winter, retreating from the dance of life to embrace the dark so that life and light may pour forth again.

This is a good place for my croning years. Here, in these rugged hills and lush valleys of the natural world, I have experienced what is true to my nature. Each season in these mountains is an invitation to learn about myself and how I might live in harmony with inner and outer energies.

In the autumn that I write this, the sparkle and fire of summer is yielding to fall's quiet, muted brilliance. It is a time of introspection, of moving deeper within, just as the sap moves down into the trunk and roots of trees.

It is a time of letting go of what no longer holds value. That's true for clothes and leaves as well as rigid attitudes. Inspired by anticipation of change in the visible world, I seek more space within—to keep what is important to me now and to release what no longer fits. Like Earth, I too must pause to reckon with the rhythms and tempos of the natural world, my own nature a reflection of her pulse.

Once, very long ago, people knew Earth as the Mother of All, feminine presence of wisdom, the Goddess, the feminine side of God. Honoring her, says Marion Woodman in *Dancing in the Flames* (p. 213), we are also

> honoring the masculine that knows her. [God and Goddess are] complimentary energies. . . .

this conscious differentiation . . . [is] essential
in order for integration (that is, wholeness) to
take place.

Into the goddess's deep caverns I have descended,
picking my way through the rubble of a life turned upside down. Mine has been a journey into the dark to find
the veins of gold, the treasure within sorrowing waiting
for me to mine it. As with a small dying, I descended
into the unknown to search for my unique essence. Like
the ancient alchemists who aimed to turn base metals
into gold, I have transmuted the everyday struggle with
illness into meaning.

The mystery is that in loss, I gain the union of the
dark and the light of my soul, and divine compassion

meets me in my deepest wound. What seems like con-
tradiction turns out to be complementary, for I bring
opposites into harmony by letting love's spark struggle
with the darkness of evil.

Now I have returned, inch by inch, to stand on Gaia's
ground and remember myself whole and holy. What is
newly born in me? What do I bring from my journey
below? There, in my darkness, in the stillness of my soul
and the pain of humility, I heard the goddess within
calling me to mercifully gather in the sufferings of body
and soul. In so doing, I discovered, like a small birthing,
the treasure of loving myself and all others from the
compassion of an open heart and the truth of my consciousness.

**Dreamlight
1998**

The world has sustained a nuclear explosion. J. and I are in a vast outdoor arena strewn with sleeping bodies. Although we were not in the vicinity of the explosion, we are inhaling toxic gasses, which have caused people to fall into a deep sleep. J. and I are among the first to awaken. Our immediate concern is to find uncontaminated water. We are told that if we exchange saliva with one another and with the other survivors, we will live. We begin to spit in one another's mouths, aware that this practice is a ritual of reverence.

This dream indicates that we all have the means to make healing possible. Its message is that healing occurs through giving one's self. To give of our essence is to give of the living water within our own bodies. Sharing from the most essential part of our selves offers compassion on a level of service, such as Mother Teresa expressed as she gathered the forsaken and afflicted into her heart.

As I emerge from my depths, a song of renewal on my lips and compassion fresh in my heart, I am surprised to discover the soft light of a new dawn shining on me. The circumstances of my life are the same. Daily, Parkinson's still challenges me. Yet all is changed. Where I am most at the mercy of unknown forces, love meets me. As though by grace, the arms of Earth are holding me as I receive the compassion of God.

The dark has taught me a keener responsiveness to the light in which what matters are life's "ordinaries"—not grandiose events but mundane happenings. Sinking my hands into the soil or listening expectantly for the song of the wood thrush, touching a hurt friend with tenderness, laughing until the tears roll down my cheeks. Life is more gentle now.

I am present to the sun as it sets in the western sky. I am present to the passion of Stravinsky's *Firebird* as the phoenix rises from ashes into new life. I am here to feel the tiny hand of a grandchild in my own, to appreciate with awe my adult children shaping their lives with integrity and authenticity. With deepened care, I find myself attending to the "Thou" before "me," as I do the work I love, with respect and recognition that each person is holy. I am here as I gaze with tenderness into the eyes of my beloved. In illness, paradoxically, I am more alive to life than ever.

Over a rough and vast wasteland, I have made my way in search of a new identity that incorporates Parkinson's as integral to my being-ness. Grappling with the realities, the challenges, and the fears of chronic illness pushed me down and down, deeply humbled—deeply enough to soften my heart and to bring forth the gift of my authentic voice. The deep feminine calls me to the words of my wisdom, experience, and the meanings I place on my life. In a process of ongoing transformation, I now hear that call and bring those words to others.

I have come home to my own nature. From my down-going, I have returned a fledgling crone. "Could it be" asks Dianne Connelly, psychologist and acupuncture practitioner, "that what widens within us forever is the ongoing act of transformation that we call love, and sometimes give other names to, like healing, wholing, and coming home?" One of my all-time favorite books is Dianne's *All Sickness is Home Sickness*. I have been homesick for me. To myself I now give mercy, for I cannot give to others what I deny myself.

I write personally of all this because writing from my inner depths brings flesh to words, restores my life, and changes me. I like calling this "transformational writing," in the words of my sister Priscilla. Like singing or dancing, painting, beading, or throwing pots, writing connects us to the archetypal energy of creation. In creating, we are created. From the world down under, I return to ask: what is your true song? What is the passion of your soul? We must find what we love and the expression that love takes in our lives.

Because of the darkness, what I see in the light is vivid, intense, and clear. Where I once spent my worldly ambition striving upward to the light, I now also know the path downward into the dark. Relaxing into a pattern of upswellings and ebbing in the natural order of things lets a more compassionate consciousness contain the

meanings of my life. It also allows love to enter—"a love,"
writes Sam Keen in *The Passionate Life*,

> that is about the task of healing. It is to practice
> the art of forgiveness and expand the circle of
> care . . . at any moment [I] may forget [my] self
> and slip into a wood thrush's song, the cry of
> an injured old man, or [my beloved's] arms. To
> love is to return to a home [I] never left, to re-
> member who [I am].

Suffering the dark now leads me to new life, and I am at
home in the skin of my soul.

ONE HUNDRED
TULIPS

The poignancy of time passing brings also the sweetness of solitude. Winter can be harsh in these mountains, lonely and dangerous. Sometimes it pinches my spirit. Engulfing the top of our mountain, gentle fog rolls silently up the gorge and settles over me. Stately pines bend as if in prayer, their branches laden with snow.

This is a time for tending the hearth of my soul, a time for listening to the silence. From within, I take on the work of befriending an aspect of my psyche I don't yet know well. As I gather the threads of my life into one weaving, fragments become heirlooms and flaws become beauty. Lines of sorrowing mark my changing face alongside wrinkles that hint of ecstasy. The wise old woman, my inner crone, is emerging from the depths of me.

Still, the optimism of youth inspirits my adventuresome nature: dreams of having babies surprise me with their frequency. Being pregnant and giving birth empowered me as woman. I felt called in that time of my life by a challenge I knew I had been created to meet. Surrendering to that process, I absorbed myself in its unfolding, day by day, until the transformation from maiden to mother was complete.

My children are now adults, yet they are still my children and will be always. As I no longer birth babies, I feel compelled to find other places to give birth to the amazing mystery of creation. For me, this is happening by writing. Both babies and stories are artistic creations, holy and amazing, inviting us into the ancient mystery of life–death–life renewal. Word by word, stories take form in a process that brings personal growth and transformation.

Writing has become crucial to my health and well being. It mobilizes archetypal creativity, which links me to a larger reality. It revitalizes me so that any new creation—a song, a poem, an essay, or a baby—is part of my ongoing process of individuating and healing. It invites me to reach for the living waters of my soul: the wellspring of love, a place of softness, vulnerability, and passion.

While one aspect of my psyche travels the murky darkness of illness with a mere thread between my fingers, another part holds a golden ball of twine that unwinds as much as necessary for me to explore the dark and find my way back to the light. Together, they create balance, for I am both light and dark. I am both hag and lover. I am ordinary, and I have my gifts. I am rageful and I am gentle. If these polarities are to value their uniqueness and resolve their diverse duality, they must meet in respectful compassion. My integration— my integrity—depends on fully accepting these opposites within my psyche. That means moving beyond the rigidity of good and evil or right and wrong. Such inflexible attitudes or judgments alienate me from myself, sever my connection with God, break the bond between Earth and spirit, and separate me from you—from the experience that we are all of one heart and soul.

We are standing on common ground—the words of an old Southern hymn sing in a timeless moment in which all that has been true, will be true, and is true now are joined together in consciousness where all opposites resolve. And we are lifted up into new wholeness.

Daily I descend, and daily I ascend. A process of all life growing and changing: transmuting and transforming as part of a larger pattern of metamorphosis. As I take

275

responsibility for experiencing and understanding the living truths of my life, I heal the split in myself. I also discover an ability to love others in partnership, with trust and truth. I find I now love with unconditional tenderness, with a divine compassion that comes from the heart of God and his Goddess.

Reaching with compassion and love to bring me to new frontiers in my personal consciousness, the feminine side of God grows and evolves. When we shine the love and light of our souls on one another, the oneness grows and transforms until we each become part of the unity of Mother/Father God.

I heard the excitement in my mother's voice over the phone recently as she read an Associated Press release about research showing that the human brain does, indeed, regenerate cells. (The long-accepted belief had been that biology allotted us a number of brain cells early in life, only to have them die off as we age.) Later, I watched a Jim Lehrer interview with one of the researchers from the Salk Institute. That doctor emphasized the hope this finding brings to patients with Alzheimer's or Parkinson's, as well as those with massive injuries to the head.

While I have learned to regard research findings with cautious joy, this is the first time I received immediate communication from my unconscious. A few hours after hearing this news, I had the following dream.

Dreamlight
1998

My husband and I return to Sherman, Texas to visit the School of Open Learning. Arriving at its verdant country setting, we find that it has been closed but is soon to reopen. Looking through the school's large, sparkling-clean windows, I see its wooden rooms empty yet clean and polished to a high sheen. I comment to J., "It all makes so much sense now."

Happy and excited to be back, we plan to stay to help with the reopening. As we walk through the beautiful rolling hills, we see the teacher now awakening from a long sleep on the grass in a wooden lean-to, which she has made from scraps of wood. I know she has been waiting for the school to reopen. It occurs to me that she is a younger version of myself.

Beside her, I see a nest filled with electric-blue bird eggs. They are very beautiful. As I walk closer to get a better look, I realize they are changing into a pan of baked yeast rolls. I am amazed and then astonished to see the rolls change into a human brain. I am filled with awe.

An old friend from our Texas years arrives unexpectedly. J. and I are delighted to see him again. I awake feeling great joy, hope, and freedom.

This dream takes place in Sherman, Texas, a college town where J. Linn and I both lived in the early 1970s. There, along with other parents who brought the best of their own resources, talents, and creativity, we helped found a school (preschool through middle school) where children could proceed at their own pace. Montessori learning tools and materials enriched the interdisciplinary curriculum, in which arts were at the core. Due to the expertise and devotion of the head teacher, parents, and students, our school prospered for eighteen years. It was a time of intense creativity, close community, and longtime commitment to friendships.

Looking through the dream's large, sparkling-clean windows is like looking through the windows of the soul and discovering this beautiful world to which we all belong. I can see and understand much more about my relationship with Parkinson's, and I can now search for the yearning behind it. What have I longed for? What do I want? For what does my soul sing?

This illness insists that I find my truth and stand beneath my truth without judgment or evaluation. With conviction and with courage, I must also find the voice to speak without fear of censure or any need to be special. At the time of early symptoms, I prayed for humility to rid me of arrogance and inflation, merely inadequate covers for my own fears. Parkinson's has literally brought me to my knees so that I move into the unknowns of my life with grief and with love woven together. From the dark, I tell my story of loss; and from the light, I am learning to rejoice moment by moment with a humble heart. I find the passion to re-image myself as larger than my disability and live with renewed joy. In this way,

I find meaning and purpose in connecting to the larger reality.

The view of lush rolling hills in my dream is unlike the scruffy, dry Texas topography of waking reality. In the dream, everyone and everything is coming alive. The buildings are sparkling clean. The teacher no longer slumbers. The feminine is conscious and aware, resting until time to begin again. Beside her is the nest of eggs. Blue is the color of robins' eggs, and the robin is the harbinger of spring. Bread rises with yeast to provide the staff of life, and the human brain regenerates. All three represent the manifestation of new life potential. The same message in different ways.

It is quite appropriate that our friend shows up as a positive masculine energy. In waking life, he transformed his own life by peeling off a mask of inauthenticity. The joy, hope, and freedom I felt in this dream have not departed. The message seems to be that as much potential for new life exists now and in the future as in the past.

I feel a new consciousness moving in me. A consciousness more deeply rooted in the dark womb of Earth, where the loamy clay out of which life once formed now absorbs my suffering. In this dark sanctuary, gestation waits patiently until new life stirs with longing for the light that ushers us into bloom.

I am at rest for the time being. For this time, I am *being* in the rest of a sacred pause. For seeing my life from inside out with new clarity, I give thanks. What dualistic thinking once separated is now merging—male and female, parent and child, love and hate, fundamentalist and libertarian, sickness and health, darkness and light, reader and writer, you and I.

Polarities dissolve their opposition into a connection of love and compassion which my body and soul can hardly bear. Pain is dissolving into love. Soul fills the sinews and cells of my flesh. Deep within my heart and body, I know we are all one in spirit. Bird eggs, yeast rolls, and the adult brain pulse with life as the divine touches my waiting heart. Without my shields, I am soft and vulnerable, bendable, fluid. I cannot remain un-changed. Misfortune broke open my heart so that I would find my deepest nature. It is pure gold.

My odyssey with Parkinson's began in conscious-ness after dreaming of two iris bulbs ripped sav-agely from the earth. As this journey has taken me to my depths, a terrible sorrowing has battered my soul while something beautiful has grown in my heart. Completing this round on my life's spiral, I honor life's potential by casting a hundred red tulip bulbs into our yard. Where they land, I plant them. Growing in the dark of winter, the first tulip of spring imagines the flower that her deepest nature calls her to be.

285

EPILOGUE

The importance of suffering will always be that it drives us toward wholeness, toward reaching the totality of the psyche, in the context of the mystery of the full experience of life. Understanding and accepting the vitality and the necessity of suffering is an agonizing, difficult task, a task that rouses our soul.

We must learn not to be afraid. We can gain new, creative, and unexpected perspectives from our suffering. We can learn that in the tears of suffering, we can find the salt of wisdom, the heart of life,

—Massimilla Harris and Bud Harris
in *Like Gold Through Fire*

COMPANIONS
ON THE
JOURNEY

A BIBLIOGRAPHY

Albom, Mitch (1997). *Tuesdays with Morrie*. New York, NY: Doubleday.

Anderson, Sherry Ruth, and Patricia Hopkins (1991). *The Feminine Face of God*. New York, NY: Bantam Books.

Angelou, Maya (1978). *Phenomenal Woman*. New York, NY: Random House.

Artress, Lauren, D. (1995). *Walking a Sacred Path*. New York, NY: Riverhead Books.

Barasch, Marc Ian (1993). *The Healing Path*. New York, NY:
    G. P. Putnam's Sons.

Borysenko, Joan (1996). *A Woman's Book of Life*. New
    York, NY: Riverhead Books.

Borysenko, Joan (1987). *Minding the Body, Mending the
    Mind*. New York, NY: Bantam Books.

Borysenko, Joan. *The Power of the Mind to Heal*. Audio
    book. Niles, IL: Nightengale Conant.

Chester, Laura (1987). *Lupus Novice*. Barrytown, NY:
    Station Hill Press.

Christ, Carol P. (1980). *Diving Deep and Surfacing*. Boston,
    MA: Beacon Press.

Connelly, Dianne M. (1986). *All Sickness Is Home Sickness*.
    Self- published.

Connelly, Dianne M. (1979). *Traditional Acupuncture: The
    Law of the Five Elements*. Self-published.

Dallett, Jane O. (1991). *Saturday's Child*. Toronto, ON, Canada: Inner City Books.

de Castillejo, Irene Claremont (1973). *Knowing Woman*. New York, NY: G. P. Putnam's Sons.

Duff, Kat (1993). *The Alchemy of Illness*. New York, NY: Bell Tower.

Duvoisin, Roger C. (1991). *Parkinson's Disease*. New York, NY: Raven Press.

Ernaux, Annie (1991). *A Woman's Story*, New York, NY: Ballantine Books.

Estes, Clarissa Pinkola (1992). *Women Who Run with the Wolves*. New York, NY: Ballantine Books.

Garfield, Patricia (1991). *The Healing Power of Dreams*. New York, NY: Simon & Schuster.

Harris, Bud (1996). *The Father Quest*. Alexander, NC: Alexander Books.

Harris, Massimilla and Bud Harris (1996). *Like Gold Through Fire*. Alexander, NC: Alexander Books.

Hay, Louise L. (1982). *Heal Your Body*. Carlsbad, CA: Hay House.

Highwater, Jamake (1977). *Anpao*. Philadelphia, PA: J. B. Lippincott.

Hollis, James (1993). *The Middle Passage*. Toronto, ON, Canada: Inner City Books.

Hollis, James (1994). *Under Saturn's Shadow*. Toronto, ON, Canada: Inner City Books.

Jamison, Kay Redfield (1996). *An Unquiet Mind*. New York, NY: Vintage Books.

Joseph, Jenny (1987). *When I Am An Old Woman I Will Wear purple*. Paper-Mache Press.

Keene, Sam (1983). *The Passionate Life*. San Francisco, CA: Harper & Row.

Keene, Sam (1970). *To a Dancing God*. New York, NY: Harper & Row.

Kidd, Sue Monk (1992). *The Dance of the Dissident Daughter*. San Francisco, CA: Harper Collins.

Kreinheder, Albert (1993). *Body and Soul*. Toronto, ON, Canada: Inner City Books.

Lamott, Anne (1994). *Bird by Bird*. New York, NY: Anchor Press.

Levine, Stephen (1984a). *A Gradual Awakening*. Garden City, NY: Anchor Press.

Levine, Stephen (1984b). *Meetings at the Edge*. Garden City, NY: Anchor Press.

Lewis, C. S. (1961). *A Grief Observed*. New York, NY: Bantam Books.

Locke, Steven and Douglas Colligan (1986). *The Healer Within*. New York, NY: Dutton.

Luke, Helen M. (1995). *The Way of Woman*. New York, NY: Doubleday.

Luke, Helen M. (1984). *The Voice Within*. New York, NY: Crossroad Publishing.

Manning, Martha (1994). *Undercurrents*. San Francisco, CA: Harper Collins.

Mato, Tataya (1994). *The Black Madonna Within*. Chicago, IL: Open Court.

Meador, Betty De Shong (1994). *Uncursing the Dark*. Wilmette, IL: Chiron Publications.

Metzger, Deena (1992). *Writing for Your Life*. San Francisco, CA: Harper Collins.

Monaghan, Patricia (1999). *The Goddess Path*. St Paul, MN: Llewellyn Publications.

Murdock, Maureen (1990). *The Heroine's Journey*. Boston, MA: Shambhala Publications.

O'Donohue, John (1997). *Anam Cara*. New York, NY: Cliff Street Books.

Paschal, Eugene (1992). *Jung to Live By*. New York, NY: Warner Books.

Perera, Silvia Brinton (1981). *Descent to the Goddess*. Toronto, ON, Canada: Inner City Books.

Preat, Jane R. (1994). *Coming to Age*. Toronto, ON, Canada: Inner City Books.

The Presbyterian Hymnal. (1990). Louisville, KY: Westminster/John Knox Press.

Price, Reynolds (1994). *A Whole New Life*. New York, NY: Antheneum.

Price, Reynolds (1999). *Letter to a Man in the Fire*. New York, NY: Scribner.

Reeve, Christopher (1998). *Still Me*. New York, NY: Random House.

Reilly, Patricia Lynn (1995). *A God Who Looks Like Me*. New York, NY: Ballantine.

Samuels, Michael (1990). *Healing with the Mind's Eye*. New York, NY: Summit Books.

Satir, Virginia; John Banmen; Jane Gerber; and Maria Gomori (1991). *The Satir Model*. Palo Alto, CA: Science and Behavior Books.

Starck, Marcia and Gynne Stern (1993). *The Dark Goddess*. Freedom, CA: Crossing Press.

Wells, Rebecca (1996). *Little Alters Everywhere*. New York, NY: Harper Perennial.

Whitmont, Edward C. (1993). *The Alchemy of Healing*. Berkeley, CA: North Atlantic Books.

Woodman, Marion (1982). *Addiction to Perfection*. Toronto, ON, Canada: Inner City Press.

Woodman, Marion (1993). *Conscious Humanity.* Toronto, ON, Canada: Inner City Press.
Woodman, Marion and Elinor Dickson (1996). *Dancing in the Flames.* Boston, MA: Shambhala Publications.